Introduction to

Physiology

for Paramedical Students

Introduction to Physiology for Paramedical Students

Reena Kaur Ruprai MD

Assistant Professor
Department of Physiology
Government Medical College
Nagpur, Maharashtra

CBS
CBS Publishers & Distributors Pvt Ltd

New Delhi • Bengaluru • Chennai • Kochi • Kolkata • Mumbai • Pune
Hyderabad • Nagpur • Patna • Vijayawada

Disclaimer

Science and technology are constantly changing fields. New research and experience broaden the scope of information and knowledge. The author has tried her best in giving information available to her while preparing the material for this book. Although, all efforts have been made to ensure optimum accuracy of the material, yet it is quite possible some errors might have been left uncorrected. The publisher, the printer and the author will not be held responsible for any inadvertent errors, omissions or inaccuracies.

Introduction to
Physiology
for Paramedical Students

ISBN: 978-81-239-2264-5

First Edition: 2013
Reprint: 2016 ; 2017

Published by Satish Kumar Jain and produced by Varun Jain for
CBS Publishers & Distributors Pvt Ltd
4819/XI Prahlad Street, 24 Ansari Road, Daryaganj, New Delhi 110 002, India.
Ph: 23289259, 23266861, 23266867 Website: www.cbspd.com
Fax: 011-23243014 e-mail: delhi@cbspd.com; cbspubs@airtelmail.in.
Corporate Office: 204 FIE, Industrial Area, Patparganj, Delhi 110 092
Ph: 4934 4934 Fax: 4934 4935 e-mail: publishing@cbspd.com

Branches

- **Bengaluru:** Seema House 2975, 17th Cross, K.R. Road, Banasankari 2nd Stage, Bengaluru 560 070, Karnataka
  Ph: +91-80-26771678/79 Fax: +91-80-26771680 e-mail: bangalore@cbspd.com
- **Chennai:** 20, West Park Road, Shenoy Nagar, Chennai 600 030, Tamil Nadu
  Ph: +91-44-26680620, 26681266 Fax: +91-44-42032115 e-mail: chennai@cbspd.com
- **Kochi:** Ashana House, No. 39/1904, A.M. Thomas Road, Valanjambalam, Ernakulam 682016, Kochi, Kerala
  Ph: +91-484-4059061-65, 67 Fax: +91-484-4059065 e-mail: kochi@cbspd.com
- **Kolkata:** 6/B, Ground Floor, Rameswar Shaw Road, Kolkata-700 014, West Bengal
  Ph: +91-33-22891126, +91-33-22891127, +91-33-22891128 e-mail: kolkata@cbspd.com
- **Mumbai:** 83-C, Dr E Moses Road, Worli, Mumbai-400018, Maharashtra
  Ph: +91-22-24902340/41 Fax: +91-22-24902342 e-mail: mumbai@cbspd.com
- **Pune:** Bhuruk Prestige, Sr. No. 52/12/2+1+3/2 Narhe, Haveli (Near Katraj-Dehu Road Bypass), Pune 411 041, Maharashtra
  Ph: +91-20-64704058, 64704059, 32342277 Fax: +91-20-24300160 e-mail: pune@cbspd.com

Representatives

- **Hyderabad** 0-9885175004
- **Nagpur** 0-9021734563
- **Patna** 0-9334159340
- **Vijayawada** 0-900066088

Printed at : Swastik Packagings, 506 F.I.E. Patparganj, Delhi -92

Preface

Introduction to Physiology for Paramedical Students is basically a concise textbook of physiology with an attempt to summarize the vast knowledge so that understanding the topic as well as reproducing will be easy.

The book is designed mainly for paramedical students but may also be a useful for last day revision by MBBS students.

The book is enriched with simple tables and flow charts. A list of questions is also given at the end of each topic for self-assessment.

Since this is the first edition, all suggestions and healthy criticism from readers will be helpful for further improvement of the book. I hope the book shall serve the purpose and help the students to learn in an easier way.

Reena Kaur Ruprai
reenakaur.ruprai@rediffmail.com

to

My father
(Late) S. Avtar Singh Kalsi
and
My father-in-low
(Late) S. Jarnail Singh Ruprai

Acknowledgements

I like a teacher who gives you something to take home to think besides homework. And a teacher gives a lot of things to take home!

Just a token of words to express my gratitude to all those people who have constantly supported me to accomplish my task:

I am grateful to Dr AS Tambe, Associate Professor, Department of Physiology, Government Medical College (GMC), Nagpur, for inspiring me to undertake this task.

My sincere thanks to Dr (Mrs) NV Mishra, Professor and Head, Department of Physiology, GMC, Nagpur, for her constant encouragement.

I am grateful to Mr YN Arjuna, CBS Publishers and Distributors, for having faith in me, and encouraging me to go ahead with the project. I am thankful to the entire editorial team for their kind cooperation and beautiful printing of the book. I am actually thankful to the publisher for giving me a break in this field.

My sincere thanks to my cherished colleagues, my juniors and seniors who had a profound influence on my personal and professional development. Without the encouragement and stimulation of such mentors work could never have been possible.

Finally, from the bottom of my heart my sincere thanks to my better-half Mr Balbir Singh Ruprai BE (Civil), MTech (Structural Engineering) who has actually designed, structurally framed and firmly constructed my words into a book form. Last but not the least, I am thankful to my angel Aamanpreet for cooperating and allowing me to do my work. I wish to say that I am honored to have both of them in my life.

Reena Kaur Ruprai
reenakaur.ruprai@rediffmail.com

Bibliography

1. Marya, RK: *Medical Physiology,* 3rd edn, CBS Publishers & Distributors, New Delhi.
2. Marya, RK: *Textbook of Physiology for Dental Students,* 2nd edn, CBS Publishers & Distributors, New Delhi.
3. Marya, RK: *Pathophysiology,* CBS Publishers & Distributors, New Delhi.
4. Marya, RK: *Learning Physiology through MCQs,* CBS Publishers & Distributors, New Delhi.
5. Chandrashekhar: *Manipal Manual of Physiology,* CBS Publishers & Distributors, New Delhi.
6. Samson Wright's *Applied Physiology,* 13th edn, Oxford Medical Publication.
7. Chatterjee, CC: Human Physiology, Vols 1 & 2, 11th edn, Medical Allied Agency.
8. Guyton, J & Hall, F: *Guyton and Hall TextBook of Medical Physiology,* 12th edn, Elsevier Publication
9. Jain, AK: *Textbook of Physiology,* Vols 1 & 2, 4th edn, Avichal Publication.
10. Khurana: *Textbook of Anatomy and Physiology for Nurses and Allied Health Sciences,* CBS Publishers & Distributors, New Delhi.
11. Khurana: *Textbook of Anatomy and Physiology for Health Professionals,* CBS Publishers & Distributors, New Delhi.

Contents

1 General Physiology

ORGANIZATION OF THE HUMAN BODY

Skin and its Appendages

Skin is the outermost covering to the human body. Its appendages include hairs, nails, sebaceous glands and sweat glands. The skin performs the following important functions:

- It acts as a physical barrier
- It plays an important role in regulating body temperature.
- It prevents loss of water from the body
- It is very important sensory organ.

Skeletal System

The basic frame work of the body is provided by a large number of bones, cartilage, ligaments, tendons, skeletal muscle that form the musculo skeletal system.

This allows the person to move to appropriate places either for obtaining food water or for protection against adverse surroundings.

Muscular System

Overlaying and usually attached to the bones are various muscles which are able to contract and relax. Three distinct types of muscles can be identified, skeletal muscles, smooth muscles and cardiac muscles.

Nervous System

Neurons are the functional unit of nervous system.

Brain and spinal cord form the central nervous system, while the peripheral nerves and ganglia constitute the peripheral nervous system. It serves important functions like regulation and coordination of body activities, learning, etc.

Cardiovascular System

The cardiovascular system consists of the heart and the blood vessels.

The circulatory system causes circulation of blood to different tissues and allows constant exchange of material between blood and interstitial fluid.

Respiratory System

The respiratory system consists of the lungs and the passages through which air reaches them. The passages are the nasal cavities, the pharynx, the trachea, the bronchi. As blood circulates to the lungs, it picks up O_2 and CO_2 diffuse from blood into the alveoli for excretion.

Gastrointestinal System

The digestive system consists of oral cavity, pharynx, oesophagus, stomach, small intestine, large intestine and other structures including liver, gall bladder and pancreas.

The system is concerned with digestion, absorption and storage of food.

Excretory System

The organ forming the excretory system is the kidney, the ureters, the bladder and the urethra. Kidney assists in maintenance of water and electrolyte balance and also helps in regulation of pH.

Reproductive System

Reproductive system is the production of a new generation of individuals of the same species. The male reproductive organs are the testis, the epididymis, the ductus deferens, the seminal vesicles, the prostrate, male urethra and the penis.

The female reproductive organs includes the ovaries, fallopian tubes, uterus, vagina, the external genitalia and the mammary glands. It performs important role in production of sperms, development of fetus, nutrition of the infant.

Endocrine system

Each endocrine gland secretes hormones which are transported to all the parts of the body in the extracellular fluid. Hormones secreting glands include pancreas, thyroid, parathyroid, adrenal, etc. Hormones regulate many activities in the body including metabolic functions of body cells, growth, reproduction, electrolyte balance.

Homeostasis

Homeostasis term was introduced by W.B. Cannon. Homeostasis means maintenance of static or constant conditions in the internal environment of cells.

Claude Bernard (1949) great French physiologist introduced the term internal environment of the body or the Millieu Interieur.

The following factors must be maintained for homeostasis as given below:

- pH
- Temperature
- Electrolyte concentrations
- Supply of O_2
- Supply of nutrients
- Hormone levels
- Metabolic end products
- Water content

Almost all systems of the body are involved in maintenance of internal environment.

The mode of operation of all the systems involved in homeostasis is through two feedback mechanism:

a. Negative
b. Positive

a. *Negative feedback mechanism:* That is in general if the activity of a particular system is increased or decreased a control system initiates a negative feedback and returns the activity towards the normal.

Examples

- When the blood pressure rises or lowers it initiates a series of reaction and returns the blood pressure to normal levels.
- When the hormone secretion is decreased or increased the feedback system returns it to normal.

b. *Positive feedback mechanism:* Positive feedback mechanism actually accelerates a process. Positive feedback mechanism is some cases is very useful.
   - Clot formation forming rupture of a vessel.
   - Child birth.

Review Questions

1. Define homeostasis
2. Write in brief how the different systems in the body help in maintaining internal environment constant. (homeostasis)
3. Write a note on positive and negative feedback mechanism.

CELL

Cell is the basic living unit of the body. The term cell was coined by Robert Hook (1665). Each cell is formed by a cell body and a membrane covering the cell body called cell membrane.

Fluid inside the cell is termed as cytoplasm. It contains minute and large dispersed particles and organelles. The clear portion of cytoplasm in which the organelles are suspended is termed as "cytosol".

Cell Membrane

The cell membrane is a protective sheath enveloping the cell body. It is also known as plasma membrane. It is a semi permeable membrane. This membrane separates the fluid outside the cell called extracellular fluid (ECF) from the fluid inside the cell called intracellular fluid (ICF).

The thickness of cell membrane varies from 70 to 100 Angstrom (Å) or 7 to 10 nm (Fig. 1.1).

Composition of Cell Membrane

The cell membrane is composed of three types of substances:
1. Proteins (55%)
2. Lipids (40%)
3. Carbohydrates (50%)

Lipids

Basic structure of a membrane is a lipid bilayer (2 molecules thick) which is continuous over the entire cell surface. This lipid

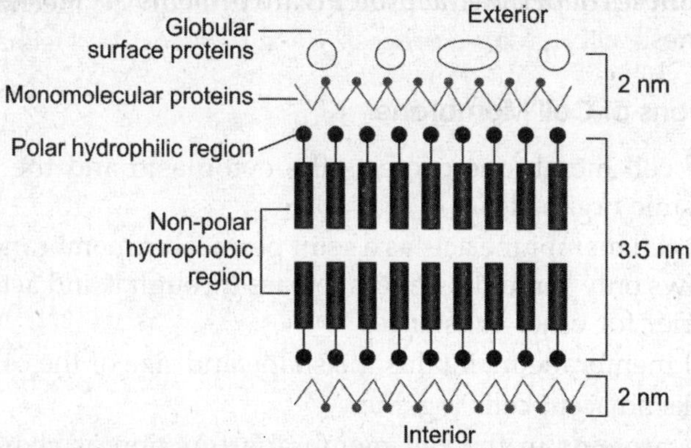

Fig. 1.1: Diagram showing structure of cell membrane

bilayer is composed of phospholipids and cholesterol. Each lipid molecule has one hydrophilic part which is soluble in water and other hydrophobic part which is soluble in lipid.

The membrane lipid is the major barrier to usual water soluble substances (e.g. urea, glucose, ions). Fat soluble substance such as alcohol, CO_2, O_2 can easily penetrate through lipid bilayer.

Proteins

Proteins of the membrane are of two types:

- Integral proteins
- Peripheral

Integral proteins

The integral proteins are the proteins that pass through the entire thickness of the cell membrane, and are highly bound to the cell membrane.

Examples of integral proteins are cell adhesion proteins, some carrier (transport) proteins, channel proteins, some hormone receptors.

Peripheral proteins

They are the proteins which are partially embedded in the center and inner surfaces of cell membrane but do not penetrate the cell membrane.

Examples of peripheral proteins are proteins of cytoskeleton enzymes.

Functions of Cell Membrane

1. The cell membrane protects the cytoplasm and the cytoplasmic organelles.
2. The cell membrane acts as a semi permeable membrane and allows only some substances to pass through it and acts as a barrier for other substances.
3. Cell membrane maintains the shape and size of the cell.
4. Links adjacent cells together.
5. The proteins in the cell membrane function as channels, pumps, carriers, enzymes, receptors.

Organelles in Cytoplasm (Fig. 1.2)

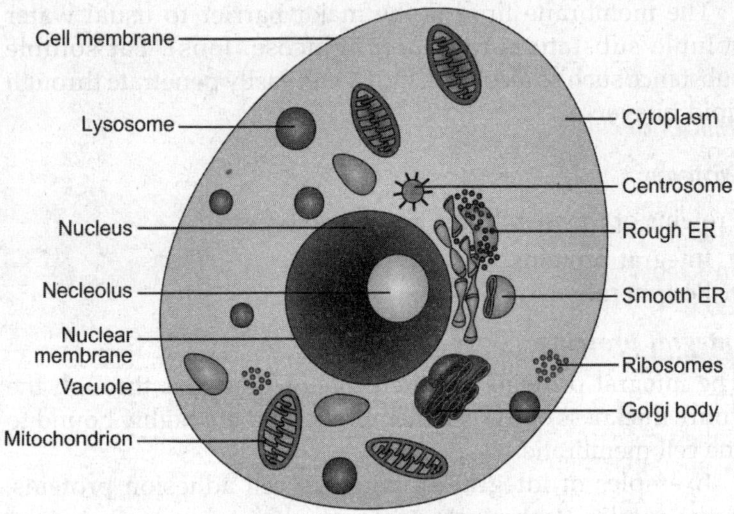

Fig. 1.2: Cell organelles

Cytoplasm organelles are the cellular structures embedded in the cytoplasm. Each organelle is having a specific function as shown in Table 1.1.

Table 1.1: Function of cell organelles

Organelles	*Functions*
Rough endoplasmic reticulum	Synthesis of proteins
Smooth endoplasmic reticulum	Synthesis of lipids and steroids.Role in cellular metabolism Catabolism and detoxification of toxic substances.
Golgi apparatus site of formation of isosomal enzymes. Transport of the material to the other part of cell.	Processing, packaging, labeling and delivery of proteins and lipids.
Lysosomes	Highly specialized intracellular digestive system. They breakdown bacteria and debris due to presence of hydrolytic enzymes.
Peroxisomes	Contains oxidases, detoxification of hydrogen peroxide and other metabolic products.
Mitochondria	Power houses of cell. Synthesis of ATP.
Ribosomes	Synthesis of protiens
Nucleus	Controls all the activities of cell synthesis of RNA. Control of cell division storage of hereditary information in genes (DNA).

Mitochondria

Mitochondria contain two layers of membrane, the outer membrane is elastic and the inner one is thrown into folds called cristae. The matrix of mitochondria contains enzymes required in Krebs cycle to produce energy which is stored in the form of ATP.

Endoplasmic Reticulum (ER)

ER it is a system of flattened membrane bound vesicular tubules called cisternae. It is of two types:

- *Rough ER:* The rough ER is characterized by the presence of ribosomes on its surface.
- *Smooth ER:* Smooth ER is devoid of ribosomes on its surfaces.

Golgi Apparatus

The golgi apparatus or golgi complex is a collection of membranous vesicles located close to the nucleus. It is continuous with endoplasmic reticulum. It is the site of concentration of proteins and completion of carbohydrate moiety of glycoproteins.

Ribosomes

Ribosomes are small spherical granules which are attached to the membrane of endoplasmic reticulum. They contain RNA and play an important role in synthesis of proteins from amino acids.

Lysosomes

Lysosomes are oval to round membrane bound organelles containing powerful digestive (hydrolytic) enzymes. They are formed by golgi apparatus.

Peroxisomes

Perioxisomes are spherical structures enclosed by a single layer of unit membrane. They contain two types of enzymes catalases and oxidases.

Centrosomes

The centrosome consists of two short cylindrical structures called centrioles. The centrioles are responsible for the movement of chromosomes during cell division.

Nucleus

Nucleus is present in all the eukaryotic cells. The nucleus consists of nuclear membrane, nucleoplasm and nucleolus.

The nucleoplasm is a gel like ground substance containing genetic material in the form of DNA.

The nucleoli are the site of synthesis of ribosomal RNA.

The nucleic acids present are mainly DNA (deoxyribonucleic acid) and RNA (ribonucleic acid).

Thus the nucleus contains genetic apparatus of the cell and ensures that on cell division each daughter cell has the necessary information to remake an exact copy of the mother cell. Thus the main function of nucleus is replication of DNA and synthesis of RNA.

Intercellular Junctions

Cells are physically joined at discrete locations along their membrane by specialized types of junctions, e.g. tight junctions, gap junctions.

Tight Junctions

They are formed when the extracellular surfaces of two plasma membranes are joined together, e.g. epithelial cells of the intestinal tract, wall of renal tubule.

Function

- Provide strength and stability to the tissues.
- Prevent ionic movement from one cell to another.

Gap Junctions

They are formed by protein channels linking the cytoplasm of adjacent cells.

Function

- Provides gap for passage of important substances like glucose, amino acid, ions, etc.
- Helps in propagation of action potential from one cell to another.

Review Questions

1. Draw a well labeled diagram showing cell and its organelles.
2. List the various cell organelles and describe the structure and function of each.
3. Write short notes on:
   a. Functions of cell membrane
   b. Intercellular junctions
   c. Structure of cell membrane

CELL TRANSPORT MECHANISM

The physiological activities of a cell depends upon the substances like nutrients, oxygen and water which must be transported into the cell and at the same time metabolic waste must be transported out of the cell.

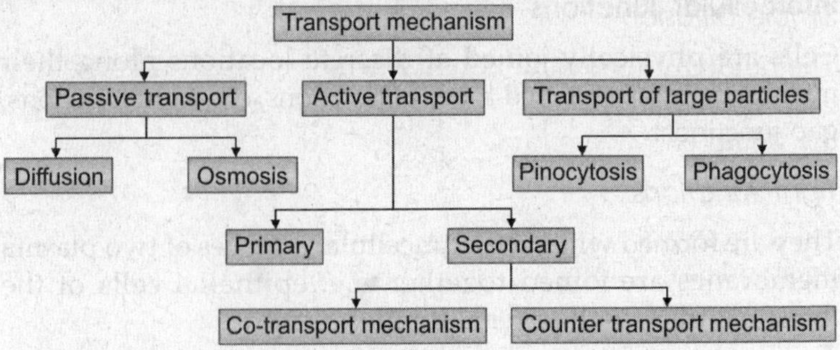

Different transport mechanism are classified as follows:

Passive Transport (Fig. 1.3)

Passive transport is the transport of a substance along the electrochemical gradient without expenditure of any energy by the cell. It includes diffusion and osmosis.

Diffusion: Diffusion is a passive process by which the molecules move from high concentration to low concentration.

It is divided into two subtypes:

1. Simple diffusion
2. Facilitated diffusion

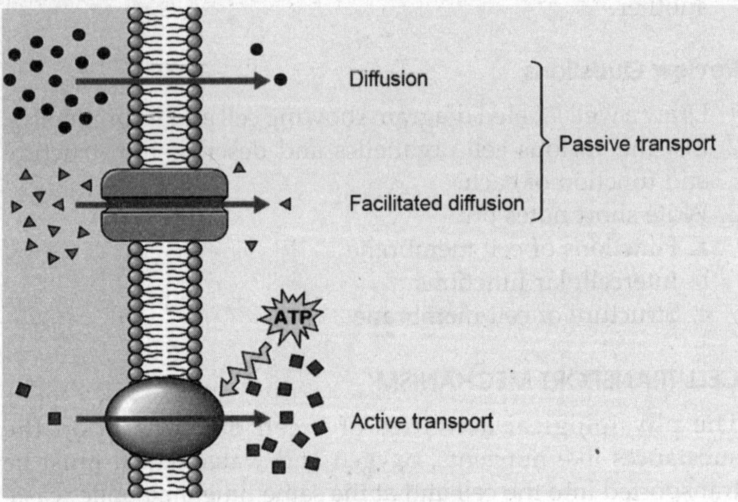

Fig. 1.3: Passive transport

Simple Diffusion

The random thermal motion of the molecules in a liquid (or a gas) that tends to redistribute themselves uniformly throughout the liquid is called simple diffusion. It occurs from higher to lower concentration and does not require a carrier.

Substances passing through the lipid bilayer of cell membrane by simple diffusion are:
- All lipid soluble substances
- Lipid soluble gases mainly CO_2, O_2, N_2.

Substances passing through protein channels of cell membrane by simple diffusion are:
- Ions mainly Na^+, K^+ and Ca^{2+}
- Water molecules

Facilitated Diffusion

It is diffusion of substances which is mediated by a carrier. The specific carrier facilitates the diffusion of a substance to the other side.

Substances that cross cell membranes by facilitated diffusion are glucose and amino acids (Fig. 1.4).

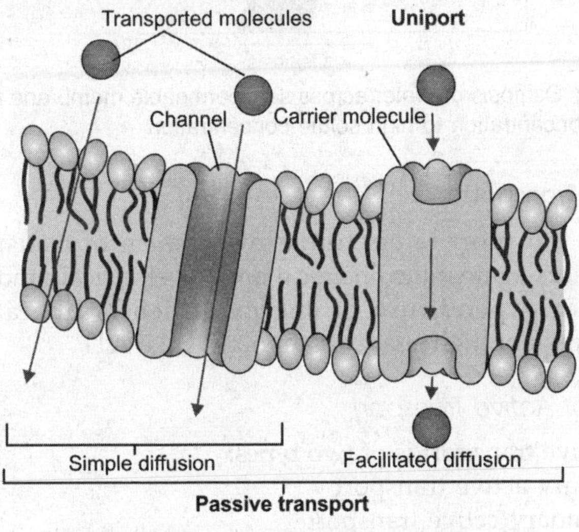

Fig. 1.4: Passive transport mechanisms

Factors affecting the rate of diffusion through cell membrane

- Thickness of the membrane
- Lipid solubility of substance
- Molecular weight of a substance
- Temperature

Osmosis

Osmosis is defined as the flow of water across a semi permeable membrane from a compartment in which the concentration of solute is lower to the one in which the concentration of solute is greater (Fig. 1.5).

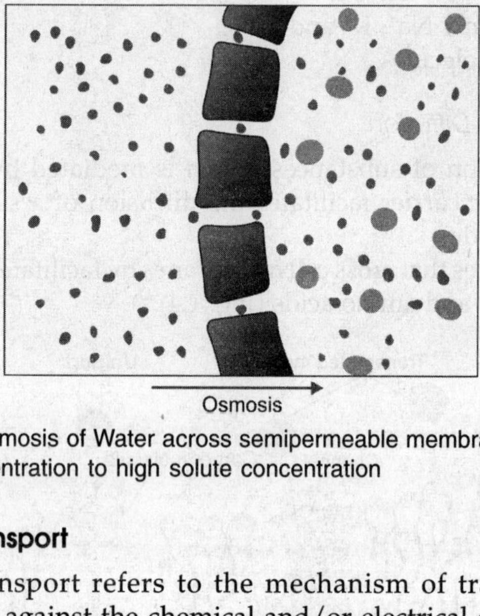

Fig. 1.5: Osmosis of Water across semipermeable membrane from low solute concentration to high solute concentration

Active Transport

Active transport refers to the mechanism of transport of substances against the chemical and/or electrical gradient. It involves expenditure of energy which is liberated by breakdown of high energy compounds like ATP.

Types of Active Transport

The active transport is of two types:

1. Primary active transport
2. Secondary active transport

Primary Active Transport

In primary active transport mechanism carrier protein in molecule possesses ATPase activity. It splits ATP molecule and obtains energy for uphill transport.

e.g. Na^+- K^+ (sodium–potassium pump)
Ca^{++} pump (Calcium pump)

Sodium–potassium (Na^+-K^+) pump/Na^+-K^+ ATPase (Fig. 1.6)

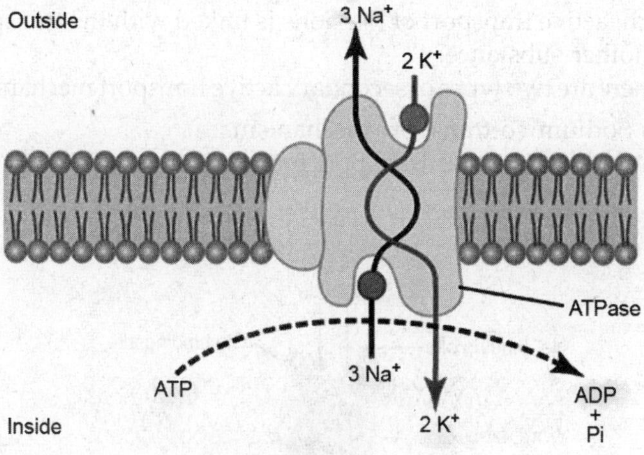

Fig. 1.6: Sodium potassium pump

It is most common pump found in all the parts of the body.

Carrier protein of this pump is made up of two globular proteins. There are three receptors sites for binding Na^+ ions on the portion of protein protruding to the interior of the cell and two receptors sites for K^+ ions on the outside surface.

Inside portion of protein also has ATPase activity.

Mechanism of action of pump

ATPase splits ATP into ADP and high-energy phosphate bond, this liberated energy causes conformational change in the protein carrier molecule which, pumps three Na^+ ions outwards and two K^+ ions inwards.

Function of Na^+-K^+ pump

- Maintains the concentration of Na^+ and K^+ ions inside and outside the cell constant.
- Maintains the cell volume.
- Na^+-K^+ pump is an electrogenic pump thus, helps in creating electrical potential across the cell membrane.

Secondary Active Transport

Secondary active transport is a type of transport process in which, active transport of Na^+ ions is linked with the transport of another substance.

There are two types of secondary active transport mechanism.

1. Sodium co-transport mechanism.
2. Sodium counter transport mechanism.

Sodium co-transport mechanism (Fig. 1.7)

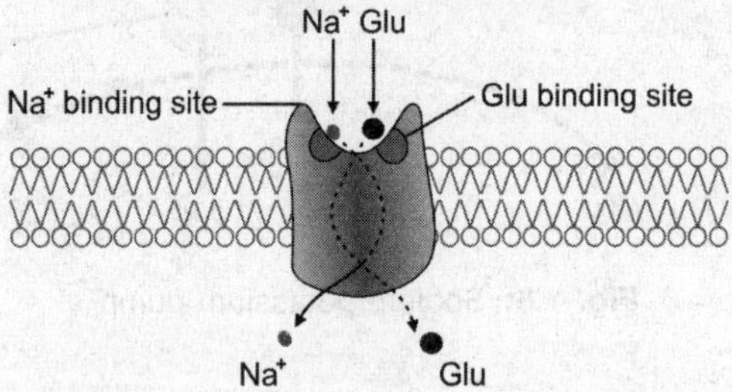

Fig. 1.7: Sodium glucose co-transport

In sodium cotransport mechanism both sodium and the substance to be transported move in the same direction, e.g. reabsorption of glucose and amino acids in the renal tubule and in the intestine.

In sodium counter transport mechanism sodium is transported in one direction and the other substance is transported in the opposite direction.

For example, Na^+-Ca^{2+} counter transport in most of the cells of the body.

Na^+-H^+ counter transport in proximal tubular cells of kidney.

Transport of large particles

Pinocytosis (cell drinking) refers to the process of engulfing liquid substances by the enfolding of cell membrane.

For example, reabsorption by renal tubular cells.

Phagocytosis (cell eating) is the process of engulfing of solid particles such as bacteria, dead tissue and foreign particles by the cells (Fig. 1.8).

For example, engulfment of bacteria by neutrophils, macrophages.

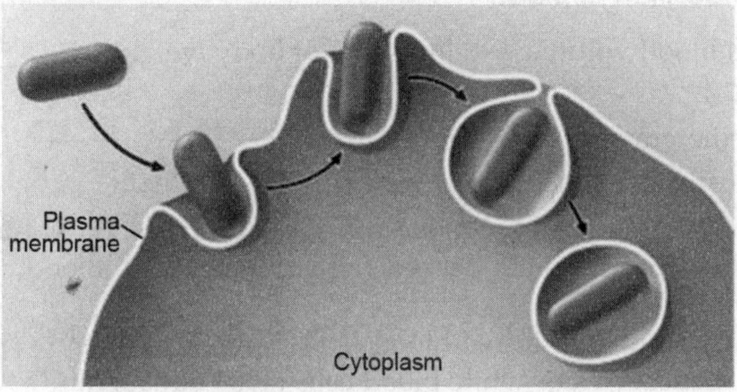

Fig. 1.8: Phagocytosis

Review Questions

1. Enumerate the different mechanisms of transport across cell membrane
2. Describe passive transport mechanism
3. Write short notes on:
   a. Primary active transport
   b. Secondary active transport
   c. Na^+ - K^+ pump

2 Blood

Blood is a specialized connective tissue in which there is liquid intercellular substance known as plasma and formed elements.

Composition of Blood

Total blood volume: 5–6 litres (8% of body weight)
pH 7.4.
Specific gravity: 1050–1060
Viscosity: 4-5 times that of water

1. Cellular elements of blood are 45% of total blood volume. They constitute the packed cell volume (PCV). Blood cells are:
   - Erythrocytes or red blood cells (5 millions/mm^3)
   - Leucocytes or white blood cells (4000–11000/mm^3)
   - Thrombocytes or platelets (1.5–4 lac/mm^3)
2. *Plasma:* 55% of blood volume (water, 91–92% and solids 8–9%)

   Solids consists of:
   a. 1% inorganic molecules
      Na^+, Ca^{2+}, Cl^- (extracellular)
      K^+, Mg^{2+}, PO_4^{3-} (intracellular)
   b. 8% organic molecules
      Plasma proteins: 6.4–8.3 gm%
      - Albumin – 3.5 gm%.
      - Globulin – 2–3 gm%.
      - Fibrinogen – 0.3 gm%.
      - Prothrombin – 40 mg%.

Non-protein nitrogenous substances including urea, uric acid, creatine, etc.

Others: Neutral fats, phospholipids, glucose and cholesterol.

Functions of Blood

1. Nutritive function.
2. Respiratory function.
3. Excretory function.
4. Protective function.
5. Transport function.
6. Maintenance of body temperature.
7. Storage function.
8. Regulation of acid base balance.
9. Regulation of water balance.

Nutritive function: Blood carries the nutritive substance like glucose, amino acids, fatty acids, vitamins, electrolytes from gut to the other tissues where they are utilized.

Respiratory function: Blood picks up oxygen from the lungs and delivers it to the tissues; also it carries away CO_2 from tissues to the lungs from where it is expelled out in the expired air.

Excretory function: Blood transports metabolic waste products such as urea, uric acid, creatinine to excretory organs (kidney, skin, intestine, lungs) for their disposal.

Protective function: Blood plays an important role in the defense mechanism of the body., e.g.

- Neutrophils and monocytes engulf the microorganism invading the body by phagocytosis.
- Lymphocytes and gamma globulins initiate immune response.

Transport function: Various hormones, antibodies are transported by the blood to the target tissue.

Maintenance of body temperature: Because of high specific heat and high conductivity blood is responsible for maintaining the balance between heat loss and heat gain in the body.

Storage function: Blood serve as a readymade source of substances stored in it (such as glucose, water, proteins, electrolytes) for use in emergency conditions like starvation, fluid loss.

Regulation of acid–base balance: Plasma proteins and hemoglobin act as buffers and helps in maintaining the acid-base balance and pH of body fluids.

Regulation of water balance: The water content of blood is freely interchangeable with the interstitial fluid and helps in maintaining the water and electrolyte balance of the body.

Plasma Proteins

Synthesis of plasma proteins: Plasma proteins mainly prothrombin, fibrinogen and albumin are synthesized only in the liver. Globulin is manufactured by reticuloendothelial cells and by lymphoid tissues.

Functions of Plasma Proteins

1. Plasma proteins (prothrombin and fibrinogen) take part in the process of blood clotting.
2. Albumin helps in maintaining colloidal osmotic pressure of blood.
3. Proteins of plasma, especially globulin due to large size and asymmetry of their structure maintain viscosity of blood, which is an important factor in maintaining blood pressure.
4. Plasma protein, fibrinogen is concerned with ESR (erythrocyte sedimentation rate). ESR is of clinical importance as a guide in prognosis of a disease.
5. Plasma proteins act as a buffer and thus help in maintaining acid–base balance.
6. Plasma proteins serve as a store house of proteins
7. Globulins play an important role in immunity.
8. Plasma proteins help in the transport of certain substances like hormones, enzymes, iron, copper, etc.

LYMPH

Lymph is a modified tissue fluid. It is the clear watery appearing fluid found in lymphatic vessels and is formed by the passage of substances from blood capillaries into tissue spaces.

Composition

Lymph is composed of:

- Water–94%
- Solids–6%
  - Proteins
  - Fats

- Carbohydrates
- Others–urea, non-protein nitrogenous substances, etc.

Functions of Lymph

- ***Nutritive:*** It supplies nutrition and oxygen to those parts of the body where blood cannot reach, e.g. cartilage.
- ***Drainage*:** It drains excess tissue fluid and metabolites and maintains the volume and composition of tissue fluid constant.
- ***Transport of proteins*:** Lymph returns proteins to the blood from the tissue spaces.
- ***Absorption of fats*:** Fats from the intestine are also absorbed through the lymphatics.
- ***Defensive:*** The lymphocyte and the monocytes of lymph act as defensive cells of the body. The lymphatic also remove bacteria from tissues.

Review Questions

1. Enumerate the functions of lymph.
2. Describe the functions of blood.
3. Composition of blood.
4. Mention the different plasma proteins and their functions.

BLOOD CELLS (Fig. 2.1)

Red Blood Cells (Erythrocytes)

Structure

a. RBC is a circular, biconcave, non-nucleated disc having diameter 7–7.2 μm.

   Advantages of biconcave disc:

   i. Allows alteration in cell volume.
   ii. Allows easy folding of RBCs while passing through the capillaries.

b. Its cell membrane contains a protein called spectrin which maintains its shape and flexibility.
c. Cell membrane contains blood group specific antigen.
d. Composition
   - RBC contains water, haemoglobin, sugar, lipid, protein, ions, enzymes of glycolytic system and carbonic anhydrase.

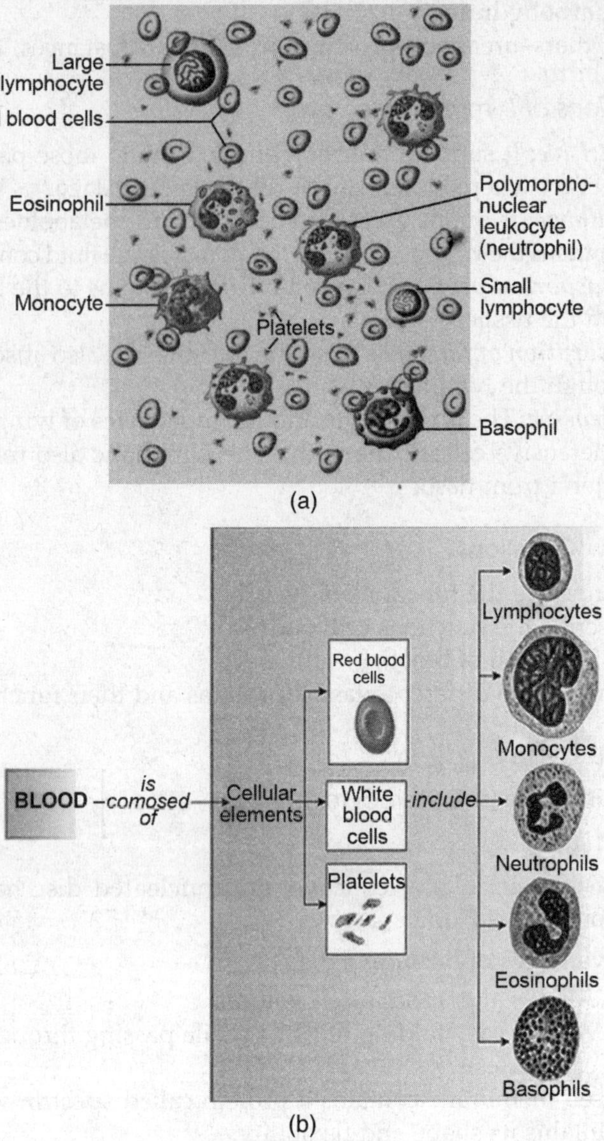

Fig. 2.1: Blood cells

e. Surface area: 140 µm²
f. Volume: 78–94 µm³

Count

i. At birth: 6–7 million/cumm
ii. Adults, Male: 5–6 million/cu mm
iii. Female: 4.5–5.5 million/cu mm

Lifespan: 120 days, after that they are destroyed by tissue macrophage system.

Functions

1. Transport of gases (CO_2 and O_2)
2. Hb in the RBCs acts as an excellent acid–base buffer.
3. Identifying blood groups.
4. Red cells help in maintaining viscosity of blood.
5. Various pigments are derived from haemoglobin after disintegration of RBC, e.g. bilirubin, biliverdin.

Erythropoiesis

1. Formation of blood cells is called hemopoiesis.
2. RBC: Erythropoiesis.
3. WBC: Leucopoiesis.
4. Platelets: Thrombopoiesis.

Site of Hemopoiesis

a. Before birth.
   - For the first two months in the yolk sac.
   - In the third month in the liver and spleen.
   - From 20th week onwards in hemopoiesis begins in the bone marrow.

b. At birth
   - Chief site is bone marrow
   - In young children active hemopoiesis occurs in both axial skeleton and bones of extremities, in adult life it is seen mainly in skull, vertebrae, ribs, pelvis and proximal ends of long bones.

Stages of Erythropoiesis (Table 2.1)

- Pronormoblast/proerythroblast
- Early normoblast
- Intermediate normoblast

Table 2.1: States of erythropoiesis

Stage	
Proerythroblast	15 – 20 μm, scanty cytoplasm, basophilic nucleus
Early normoblast	12 – 16 μm, scanty cytoplasm, large nucleus, Hb absent, mitosis present
Intermediate normoblast	10–14 μm, polychromatic cytoplasm, Nucleus condensed, Hb appears in this stage.
Late normoblast	8–10 μm, nucleus small, Hb increase in amount. Mitosis absent
Reticulocyte	7–7.5 μm, nucleus absent, Hb in the amount as in mature

- Late normoblast
- Reticulocyte
- Mature red blood cell

Mature RBC

Reticulocytes are juvenile RBC, which ultimately mature into red blood cells. Mature RBCs are devoid of nucleus, 7–7.2 μm in size.

It takes 7 days for the formation and maturation of red blood cells.

Regulation of Erythropoiesis

General Factors

Diet: Food containing essential amino acids for globin part of Hb.

Hypoxia: Stimulates bone marrow, e.g. high altitude.

Erythropoietin: Secreted by the kidneys promotes erythropoiesis.

Vitamins: Vitamin C, D deficiency can lead to anemia.

Maturation Factors

- *Metals:* Iron, copper, manganese, cobalt, vitamin C, vitamin B_{12}, folic acid, pyrodoxine.
- Intrinsic factor secreted by parietal cells of stomach which is essential for absorption of vitamin B_{12}.
- Folic acid and B_{12} are required for synthesis of DNA and maturation of nucleus.

Anaemia

Definition

Anemia is defined as decrease in oxygen carrying capacity of blood due to decrease in amount of Hb or RBC or both, below the normal range for the age and sex of the subject. (RBC count<4 million/cumm or their content of hemoglobin<12 gm%.)

Classification

1. ***Nutritional/deficiency anaemia:*** Iron deficiency anaemia, megaloblastic anemia (vitamin B_{12} and folic acid deficiency)
2. ***Blood loss/haemorrhagic anaemia:*** GIT bleeding: ulcer, haemorrhoids.

Renal tract: Hematuria, in females; excessive menstruation, post-menopausal bleeding.

3. ***Hemolytic anaemia***
   - Sickle cell disease.
   - Hereditary spherocytosis.
4. ***Aplastic anaemia***
   - Non functioning marrow, exposure to heavy metals, X-rays, radiations.
   - Anaemia due to chronic diseases like tuberculosis, malignancy.

Morphological anaemia

1. *Normocytic normochromic:* Aplastic anemia.
2. *Microcytic hypochromic:* Iron deficiency anemia.
3. *Macrocytic normochromic:* Megaloblastic anemia.

Polycythemia

Increase in RBC count >6 million/cu mm.

Causes

Physiological

i. At birth
ii. High altitude

Pathological

i. Congenital heart disease
ii. Dehydration

iii. Shock
iv. Tumor of bone marrow, polycythemia vera.

Haemoglobin

- Haemoglobin is the red, oxygen carrying pigment in the RBCs.
- It consists of protein globin and iron containing pigment called haem.
- Globin is made up of 4 polypeptide chains, 2α and 2β.
- Normal values:
  At birth: 23 gm/dl
  Adults:
  Male: 14–18 gm/dl
  Female: 12–15.5 gm/dl

Adult Haemoglobin (HbA)

It is of two types:
1. Haemoglobin A ($a2\ \beta_2$)
2. Haemoglobin A_2 ($\alpha_2\ \delta_2$)

Functions of Haemoglobin

1. Haemoglobin is essential for oxygen carriage.
2. It plays an important role in CO_2 transport.
3. It constitutes one of the important buffer of blood and helps to maintain acid–base balance.
4. Various pigments are formed after disintegration of haemoglobin (bilirubin, biliverdin, etc.).

Granulocytes

White blood cells (leucocytes) are the nucleated elements of blood which play a very important role in the defense mechanism of the body.

Classification

A. **Granulocytes, i.e. WBCs with granules in the cytoplasm**
- Neutrophils 50–70%
- Eosinophils 1–4%
- Basophils <1%

B. **Agranulocytes, i.e. WBCs without granules in the cytoplasm.**
- Lymphocytes 20–40%
- Monocytes 2–8%

Total Leucocyte Count (TLC)
At birth: 20,000/cu mm
Adults : 4-11,000/cu mm

Leucopenia: Decrease in TLC below 4,000/cu mm

Causes
- Starvation
- Typhoid fever
- Viral fever
- Bone marrow depression.

Leucocytosis: Increase in TLC >11,000/cu mm

Causes
- Newborn
- Exercise
- Stress
- Pregnancy
- Menstruation, lactation
- Pyogenic infections

Leukaemia

It is a cancerous condition where the WBC count is >50,000/ cu mm and immature cells are present in blood.

Functions of WBC

1. ***Phagocytosis:*** The neutrophils and the monocytes engulf the bacteria and foreign particles and digest them, this process is called phagocytosis.
2. ***Antibody formation:*** Lymphocytes manufacture immunoglobulins and plays an important role in defensive mechanism of the body.
3. ***Secretion of heparin:*** Basophils secrete heparin which prevents intravascular clotting.
4. ***Antihistamine function:*** Eosinophils are rich in histamine which is believed to defend against allergic conditions.

5. ***Manufacture of trephones:*** Leucocytes synthesize certain substances called trephones from plasma proteins which exert influence on nutrition, growth and repair of tissues.

Structure of WBC

Neutrophils

- 10-14 µm in size.
- Multilobed purple coloured nucleus.
- Fine granules present in the cytoplasm.

Functions

Primary function of neutrophil is to provide the first line of defense against invading microorganisms by phagocytosis. The enzymes present in the neutrophilic granules digest the bacteria.

Increase in neutrophil (**neutrophilia**) is seen in:
- Pregnancy, menstruation, stress.
- Bacterial infections.

Eosinophils

Structure

- 10-14 m in size.
- Purple coloured nucleus.
- Acidophilic cytoplasm.
- With course granules (bright red).

Functions

- Eosinophils are concerned with inhibition of allergic conditions.
- They also attack parasites.

Rise in count (**eosinophilia**) is seen in.
- Allergic conditions like asthma, parasitic infestations.

Basophils

Structure

- 10-14 m in size.
- Purple coloured nucleus.
- Basophilic cytoplasm with coarse granules (blue or purple).

Functions

- Basophils secrete histamine which mediates anaphylactic reactions.
- They also secrete heparin which acts as an anticoagulant.

Basophilia is seen in chronic lymphoid leukaemia.

Lymphocytes

Structure

There are two types of lymphocytes
1. Small lymphocyte: 7–10 μm.
2. Large lymphocyte: 10–14 μm.

Single, big, purple coloured nucleus.
Cytoplasm pale blue with no granules.

Functions

Lymphocytes provide cellular (T lymphocytes) and humoral (B lymphocytes) immunity.

Lymphocytosis is seen in chronic infections like tuberculosis, viral infections.

Monocytes

Structure

- 10-14 μ in size.
- Pale nucleus
- Pale blue cytoplasm with no granules.

Functions

- Monocytes are the second line of defense in the body.
- **Monocytosis** is seen in kala azar, infectious mononucleosis.
- Development of white blood cells.

Leucopoiesis

- Granulocytes develop mainly in the bone marrow.
- Stages of development of granulocytes are as follows:

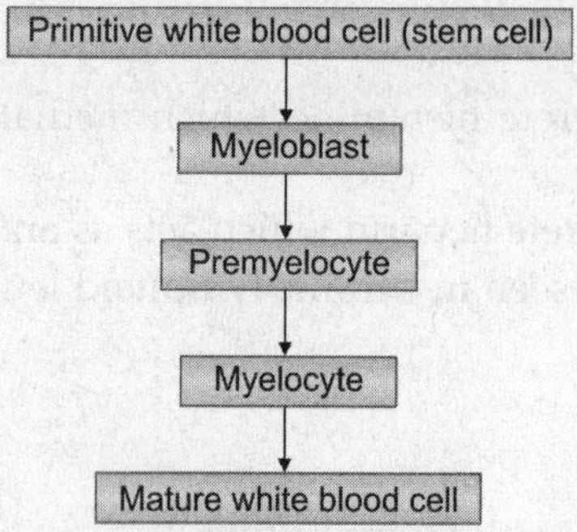

Agranulocytes develop in the bone marrow but mainly in the lymphoid tissues (thymus, spleen, lymph nodes, etc.)

Platelets

Platelets or thrombocytes are small colourless non nucleated refractile bodies, 2–4 μm in diameter. Its cytoplasm has following active factors:

- Contractile proteins like actin and myosin.
- Endoplasmic reticulum, Golgi apparatus, mitochondria
- Prostaglandins
- Fibrin stabilizing factor, which plays an important role in blood coagulation.
- Growth factor. This causes growth of fibroblast, and helps in repair of damaged vessel wall.
- Von Willebrand's factor which helps in adherence of platelets.
- ATP, ADP, 5-hydroxytryptamine (serotonin) [5-HT].

Development of Platelets

The platelets are formed from megakaryocytes in the bone marrow; development of platelets is called thrombopoiesis.

Lifespan

Lifespan of platelets varies from 8 to 12 day. Platelets are destroyed by tissue macrophage system in spleen.

Normal Count and Variation

Normal platelets count ranges from 1,50,000 to 4,50,000/cu mm.

Physiological Variation

Platelets count may increase after severe muscular exercise and at high altitudes.

Pathological Variation

Thrombocytosis (increase in the platelet count) occurs after:

1. Splenectomy
2. Haemorrhage
3. Major surgical operation.

Thrombocytopenia (decrease in the platelet count)

- Idiopathic thrombocytopenic purpura.
- Bone marrow depression.
- Viral infections, e.g. dengue fever.
- Hypersplenism.

Function of Platelets

Platelets perform following functions:

1. ***Role in haemostasis:*** Haemostasis refers to spontaneous arrest of bleeding from an injured blood vessel. Platelets play following role in haemostasis:
   - *Vasoconstriction:* Platelets secrete serotonin (5-HT) which cause vasoconstriction of blood vessel.
   - Haemostatic plug is formed by platelets due to their property of adhesiveness and aggregation.
   - Platelets repair the vascular opening by formation of plug.
2. ***Role of clot formation:*** When blood is shed, the platelets disintegrate and liberate thromboplastin which activates prothrombin into thrombin and thus initiates blood clotting.
3. ***Clot retraction:*** Contraction of contractile proteins (actin, myosin) present in the platelets play an important role in clot retraction.
4. ***Role in defense mechanism:*** Platelets due to their property of agglutination are capable of phagocytosis.
5. ***5-HT,*** present in the platelets help in haemostatic mechanism.
6. Platelets also help in the **repair of capillary endothelium**.

Purpura

Purpura is a disease in which there is decrease in the number of platelets in the blood. Haemorrhage occurs beneath the skin and mucous membrane. The clotting time remains normal but the bleeding time is prolonged and the clot does not retract.

Blood Groups

- **Agglutinogens**, refers to antigens present on cell membrane of RBC.
- **Agglutinins**, refers to antibody against agglutinogens present in the plasma.
- Depending upon the type of antigen present or absent on the cell membrane of RBC, various blood group systems are known.

Major Blood Group System

1. Classical ABO
2. Rh blood group.

Minor Blood Group System

1. MNS
2. Lewis, duffy, kell, etc.

Landsteiner Law

Karl Landsteiner in 1900 framed this law which states that

1. If an antigen is present on the RBC of an individual, the corresponding antibody must be absent from the plasma.
2. If an antigen is absent on the RBC of an individual, the corresponding antibody must be present in the plasma.
3. This law is applicable only to ABO blood group system.

Classical Blood Group System

The individuals are divided into four major blood groups depending upon the presence or absence in their RBCs membrane of the blood group specific antigen A,B,O (Table 2.2).

Table 2.2: Classical blood group system

Blood group	*Agglutinogens present in RBC*	*Agglutinins present in serum*
O	nil	α and β
A	A	β
B	B	α
AB	AB	Neither α nor β (nil)

Blood group A

Antigen A present on the RBC cell membrane, and anti-B (β) antibody present in the plasma.

Blood group B

Antigen B present on the RBC and anti-A (α) antibody present in plasma.

Blood Group AB

Antigen present on RBC membrane is both A and B and no antibodies are present in the plasma.

Blood Group O

Absence of any antigen on RBC and presence of both α and β in the plasma.

Rh (Rhesus) Blood Group

The antigen responsible for this blood group system is called Rh antigen or Rh factor. The Rh antigen is 'D' and its antibody is called anti-D.

If the Rh antigen is present, individuals are Rh positive (85%), if the Rh antigen is absent then the individual is Rh negative.

The Rh factor was discovered by Landsteiner and Weiner in 1940.

Rh Factor and Hemolytic Disease *(Erythroblastosis foetalis)*

If mother is Rh negative and fetus is Rh positive, the mother responds by forming anti-D which returns to fetal circulation and tends to destroy fetal RBCs.

Since sensitization occurs generally at birth, first child is normal. It can be prevented by giving a single dose of anti-Rh antibodies to mother soon after child birth.

Uses of blood grouping tests

- In the blood transfusion.
- In pregnancy (Rh incompatibility).
- Investigation of paternity disputes.
- Medicolegal investigations.

Blood Transfusion

1. Group A and group B can safely receive blood from their own group and group O.
2. Persons of blood group AB have no circulating antibodies and can therefore be given blood of any type, **universal recipient**.
3. Persons of blood group O contain no antigens and their blood can be given to anyone, **universal donors.**

Cross Matching

It is to match the serum of the recipient directly against the RBCs of the donor and again to match the RBCs of the recipient against the serum of the donor, if there is agglutination in either case it indicates incompatibility.

Indications of Blood Tansfusion

1. Blood loss, accidents, and major operations.
2. Exchange transfusion
3. Bleeding disorders like, aplastic anaemia, hemophilia, hemolytic anaemia.
4. Acute poisoning, carbon monoxide poisoning.

Complications of Blood Transfusion

1. In apparent hemolysis.
2. Post transfusion hemolytic jaundice.
3. Mechanical over loading of circulation.
4. Transmission of diseases; AIDS, hepatitis, malaria.
5. Pyrogenic infections.
6. Allergic reactions.

IMMUNITY

Capacity of human body to resist all types of microorganisms and their toxins is called immunity.

Classification of Immunity

Immunity is classified as:
1. Innate (natural) immunity.
2. Acquired immunity.

Innate Immunity

It is the inborn capacity of the body to offer resistance to pathogens and their products. It is also known as **non specific** immunity.

Innate immunity is provided by the following mechanisms:
- Mechanical barrier against invading microorganisms, e.g. skin, mucosa.
- Secretions (sweat, salivary, lacrimal), gastric juice, tears contain antibacterial substances.
- Cough reflex, sneeze reflex.
- Interferon, natural killer cells, phagocytes (neutrophils, monocytes).

Acquired Immunity

The resistance that an individual acquires during lifetime is known as acquired immunity.
- Cell mediated (cellular) immunity: It is mediated by **T lymphocytes**.
- Antibody mediated (Humoral) immunity: It is mediated by **B lymphocytes**.

Cell Mediated Immunity

It is mediated by T cells. T cells are of following types:
- Helper T cells (CD4+ T cells).
- Cytotoxic T cells(CD8+ T cells).
- Suppressor T cells.
- Helper T cells are involved in the regulation of antibody formation by B lymphocytes.
- Cytotoxic T cells kills cancer cells, virus infected cells and transplanted cells.
- Suppressor T cells inhibit the function of both B cells and T cells.

Antibody Mediated Immunity

Antibody mediated immunity is brought about by B cells.

B cells produce antibodies and destroy the antigens by various mechanisms as follows:

- By neutralizing the antigens
- By precipitation
- By lysis.

Antibodies

Antibody is a protein called immunoglobulin. They are synthesized by B lymphocytes. They classified as following:

1. IgM 2. IgA 3. IgG
4. IgD 5. IgE

Mechanism of Action of Immunoglobulin

Immunoglobulin act by:

- Agglutination
- Precipitation
- Neutralization
- Lysis

AIDS (Acquired Immunodeficiency Syndrome)

AIDS is caused by **HIV** (human immunodeficiency virus). It specifically attacks the helper T cells. Without adequate number of T cells, the B lymphocytes cannot form antibodies and the cytotoxic T cells also cannot function properly. Thus the patient suffering from AIDS develops cancer or infections.

It is transmitted by unprotected sexual intercourse with an infected partner, contaminated blood or blood products from one person to another and also from infected mother to baby.

Passive Immunity

Direct transfer of preformed antibodies from one person to another is called passive immunity.

For example from mother to fetus, vaccination, etc.

Blood Coagulation

Blood Clotting Factors

i.	Factor	I	Fibrinogen.
ii.	Factor	II	Prothrombin.
iii.	Factor	III	Thromboplastin.
iv.	Factor	IV	Calcium.
v.	Factor	V	Labile factor.

vi. Factor ——
vii. Factor VII Proconvertin.
viii. Factor VIII Antihemophilic factor.
ix. Factor IX Christmas factor.
x. Factor X Stuart factor.
xi. Factor XI Plasma thromboplastin antecedent (PTA).
xii. Factor XII Hageman factor.
xiii. Factor XIII Fibrin stabilizing factor.

Steps in Coagulation

1. ***Formation of prothrombin activator:*** Prothrombin activator is a complex which is formed when there is damage to the vessel wall.
2. ***Conversion of prothrombin to thrombin:*** Prothrombin activator formed converts prothrombin to thrombin.
3. ***Conversion of fibrinogen to fibrin:*** Thrombin acts as an enzyme and converts soluble fibrinogen to insoluble fibrin threads. These fibrin threads form the meshwork in which blood cells are entangled.

There are two pathways of coagulation:
1. **Intrinsic pathway** (Fig. 2.2)
2. **Extrinsic pathway** (Fig. 2.3)

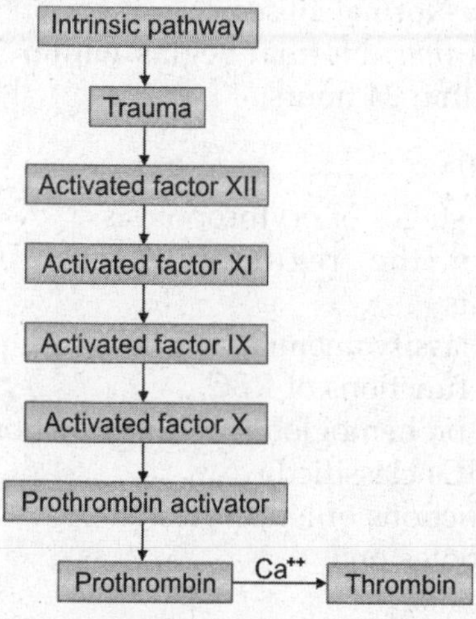

Fig. 2.2: Schematic diagram of intrinsic pathway

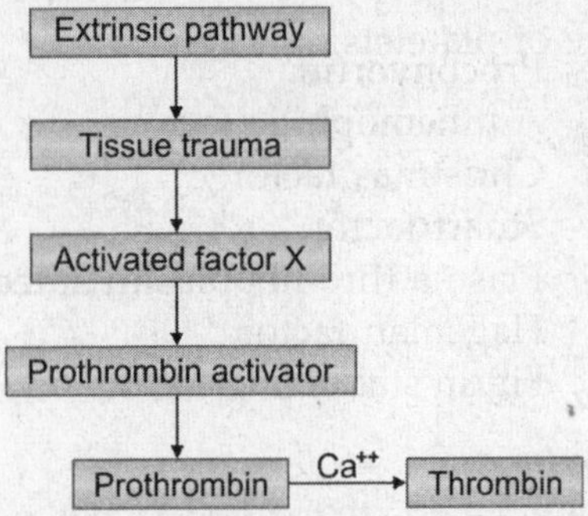

Fig. 2.3: Schematic diagram of extrinsic pathway

Hemophilia

Hemophilia is a disorder in which clotting time is prolonged. It is caused by deficiency of **Factor VIII**. It is an inherited sex-linked recessive anomaly due to an abnormal gene on X- chromosome. Therefore, females do not suffer, they are carriers and males manifest the disease.

Laboratory tests in clotting disorders

1. *Coagulation time:* Normal 3–6 min.
2. *Prothrombin time:* Normal 11–16 sec.
3. *Partial thromboplastin time:* Normal 40 sec.
4. *Thrombin time:* Normal 10 sec.
5. *Clot retraction time:* Normal begins within 2 hours and is completed within 24 hours.

Review Questions

1. Describe the stages of erythropoiesis.
2. Write down the regulation/factors required for erythropoiesis.
3. Define and classify anemia.
4. Mention the functions of RBC.
5. Write a note on hemoglobin and its functions.
6. How are WBCs classified.
7. Write the functions of leucocytes.
8. Write short notes on:
   a. Polycythemia.
   b. Leucocytosis.

c. Structure of platelets.
d. Extrinsic and intrinsic pathway of clotting.
e. Immunity.
f. Hemophilia.
g. AIDS.
h. Antibody mediated immunity.
i. T cell mediated immunity.
j. Immunoglobulin.
k. Innate immunity.

9. Describe in brief the functions of platelets. What is purpura?
10. Enumerate the clotting factors.
11. Describe in brief the process of clot formation.
12. What are the different types of immunity.

3 Nerve Muscle

NEURON (Fig 3.1)

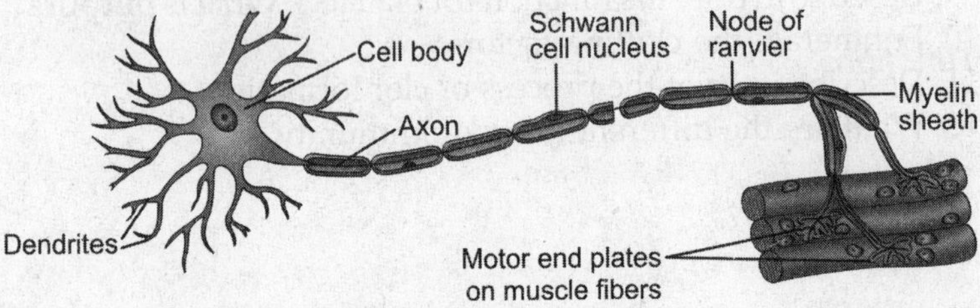

Fig. 3.1: Motor neuron

Relays messages from the brain or spinal cord to the muscles and organs.

Neuron, or the nerve cell is defined as the structural and functional unit of the nervous system.

The nervous system is made up of neurons more than 10^{12} neurons.

Structure: Each neuron is made of three parts:
1. Nerve cell body.
2. Dendrite.
3. Axon.

Nerve Cell Body

The cell body of a neuron is also called the soma or perikaryon. It is constituted by a mass of cytoplasm called neuroplasm covered by a cell membrane.

The cytoplasm contains a large nucleus, Nissl bodies, neurofibrils, mitochondria and golgi apparatus.

Centrosome is absent in the nerve cell body due to which it has no ability of cell division.

Dendrites

The dendrites are multiple small branched processes. They are the receptive processes of the neuron receiving signals from other neurons.

Axon

The axon is the single longer process of the nerve cell.

The axon terminates by dividing into a number of branches, each of them ends into synaptic knobs.

Functions

Nerve cell body

- It maintains the functional and anatomical integrity of the axon.
- Synthesizes proteins which are associated with neurotransmitters.

Dendrites

It is transmits the impulses towards the cell body.

Axon

It propagates and transmits propagated impulses away from the cell body.

Synaptic knobs

Stores and release the chemical neurotransmitter (acetylcholine).

Non myelinated nerve fibre

The nerve fibres which are not covered by myelin sheath are called non myelinated nerve fibres.

Myelinated nerve fibre

The nerve fibres which are insulated by myelin sheath are called myelinated nerve fibres.

Myelin Sheath

Myelin sheath is a thick lipoprotein sheath. It is not continuous but absent at regular intervals. The area where the myelin sheath is absent is called node of ranvier.

The formation of myelin sheath around the axon is called myelinogenesis. It is formed by Schwann cells.

Function of Myelin Sheath

- Myelin sheath is responsible for faster conduction of impulse through the nerve fibres.
- Myelin sheath has a high insulating capacity because of this it restricts the impulse within a single nerve fibre and prevents stimulation of neighbouring nerve fibres.

Neurotrophins

- Neurotrophins are the protein substances which play an important role in growth and function of nervous tissue, e.g.
- Nerve growth factor.
- Brain derived neurotrophic growth factor.
- Fibroblast growth factor.

Classification of Nerve Fibre

Nerve fibres can be classified in different ways as follows:
1. Myelinated and nonmyelinated.
2. Somatic and visceral.
3. Motor and sensory.
4. Erangler and Gasser's classification (Table 3.1).
5. Physioclinical classification (Table 3.2).

Table 3.1 : Erangler and Gasser's classification

Nerve fibre	*Type*	*Diameter*	*Conduction velocity*
1. Myelinated	A α β γ δ	12–20 μm	70–120 m/sec
2. Myelinated	B	>3 μm	4–30 m/sec
3. Unmyelinated	C	0.4–1.2 μm	0.5–4 m/sec

Table 3.2: Physioclinical classification

1. Sensitivity to hypoxia	B-fibres
2. Sensitivity to pressure	A-fibres
3. Sensitivity to local anaesthetics	C-fibres

Properties of Nerve Fibre

- Excitability.
- Conductivity.
- Refractory period.
- Adaptation.
- All or none law.

Excitability

Excitability is that property of the nerve fibre by virtue of which it responds to a suitable stimulus by generating a nerve signal.

Stimulus

Stimulus is defined as any change in the external environment that elicits response from excitable tissue.

Types of stimuli

- Thermal.
- Electrical.
- Mechanical.
- Chemical.

Action Potential or Nerve Impulse

The action potential is defined as the brief sequence of changes which occur in the resting membrane potential when stimulated by a threshold stimulus (Fig. 3.2).

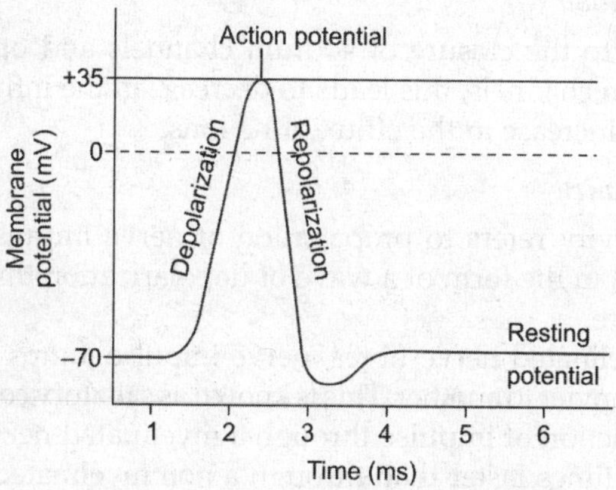

Fig. 3.2: Action potential of nerve fibre

- Phases of action potential.
- Depolarization.
- Repolarization.

Under resting condition nerve fibre has got resting membrane potential of –70 mV. This is called polarized state.

1. When the nerve is stimulated, there is a brief deflection of baseline, the **stimulus artifact.**
2. The stimulus artifact is followed by a latent period of 0.5–1 ms.
3. The first manifestation of the approaching impulse is beginning of depolarization. At this time potential at the site rises abruptly from –70 mV to +35 mV.
4. After reaching +35 mV, the phase of depolarization is completed and repolarization begins.

Ionic basis of Action Potential (Hodgkin –Huxley Theory)

Polarization

Resting membrane potential is negative at rest (–70 mV) due to selective permeability of membrane and distribution of cations (Na^+) outside and anions (K^+) inside.

Depolarization

It is due to opening of voltage gated sodium channels and increase in the permeability of Na^+ ions, with influx of Na^+ ions.

Repolarization

It is due to the closure of sodium channels and opening of potassium channels, this leads to decrease in the influx of Na^+ ions and increase in the efflux of K^+ ions.

Conductivity

Conductivity refers to propagation of nerve impulse (action potential) in the form of a wave of depolarization through the nerve fibre.

In myelinated nerve fibres, nerve impulse jumps from one node of ranvier to another. This is known as saltatory conduction.

Conduction of impulse through a myelinated nerve fibre is about 50 times faster than through a non myelinated fibre.

Refractory period

Refractory period is the period in which the nerve fibre does not give any response to a stimulus.

Refractory period are of two types:

1. Absolute refractory period.
2. Relative refractory period.

1. *Absolute refractory period:* Absolute refractory period is the period during which the nerve does not show any response at all, whatever may be the strength of stimulus.
2. *Relative refractory period:* Relative refractory period is the period during which the nerve fibre shows response, if the strength of the stimulus is increased to maximum.

All-or-none law

Action potential in the nerve fibre obeys all-or-none law, which states that when a nerve fibre is stimulated either it gives a maximum response, or does not give response at all.

Adaptation

While stimulating a nerve fibre continuously the excitability of the nerve is greater in the beginning. Later the response decreases slowly and finally the nerve does not show any response at all. This phenomenon is known as adaption.

Review Questions

1. Draw a well labeled diagram of neuron
2. Enumerate the properties of nerve fibre.
3. Classify nerve fibres
4. Describe the action potential of nerve fibre with ionic basis of different phases.

NEUROMUSCULAR JUNCTION

Neuromuscular/myoneural junction is the junction between the motor nerve fibre and skeletal muscle fibre (Fig. 3.3).

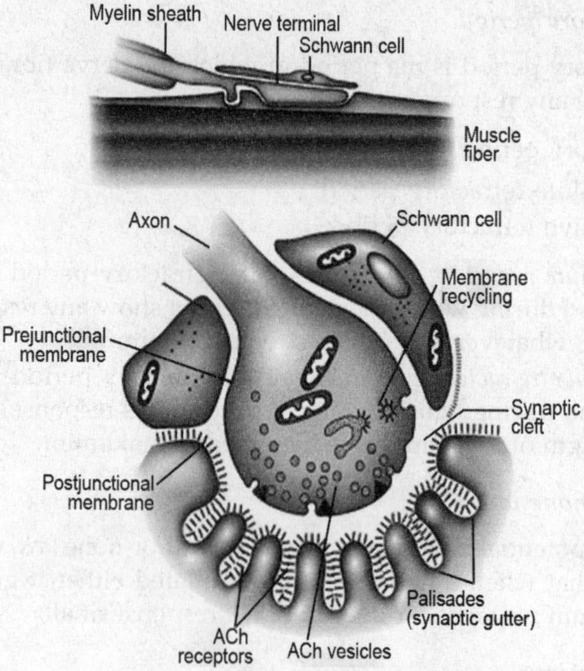

Fig. 3.3: Neuromuscular Junction

Structure

The axon of a neuron supplying a skeletal muscle loses its myelin sheath and divides into number of fine branches which ends in small swellings called synaptic knobs which form neuromuscular junction, at the centre of muscle fibre (motor end plate). The synaptic knob has vesicles containing acetyl choline, responsible for synaptic transmission.

Presynaptic Membrane

This refers to the axonal membrane.

Postsynaptic Membrane

This is the name given to the muscle fibre membrane in the region neuromuscular junction. It is thrown into folds called Palisades, which increase the surface area on which the neurotransmitter can act.

Synaptic Cleft

It is 50–100 nm wide space between the presynaptic and postsynaptic membrane.

Neuromuscular Transmission

The neuromuscular junction transmits the impulses from the nerve to muscle. The sequence of events which causes transmission of impulse through neuromuscular junction are:

- Release of acetyl choline by nerve terminals.
- Effect of acetyl choline on post synaptic membrane.
- Development of end plate potential.
- Removal of acetyl choline by cholinesterases.
- Initiation of the action potential in muscle fibre.

When the nerve impulse (action potential) reaches the presynaptic membrane acetyl choline is released by exocytosis.

The acetyl choline so released diffuses in the synaptic cleft and binds to ACh receptors leading to opening up of the ACh gated sodium channel.

Large number of Na^+ ions from the ECF enters inside the muscle fibre cause depolarization of post synaptic membrane creating the end plate potential.

The resting membrane potential in skeletal muscle membrane is –90 mV, when the end plate potential reaches a threshold of –30 to –40 mV it leads to the development of action potential in the muscle fibre.

The ACh released in the synaptic cleft is removed within one millisecond by the enzyme acetyl cholinesterase, which results in repolarization of the membrane. Removal of ACh prevents repeated excitation of muscle fibre.

Myasthenia Gravis

It is an autoimmune disease caused by formation of antibodies against the acetyl choline receptors.

The disease is characterized by rapid onset of fatigue and generalized muscular weakness.The most commonly involved muscles are extraocular, facial, swallowing and mastication muscles.

MUSCLE

There are more than 600 muscles in our body. Muscles perform many useful functions which help us in doing daily activities.

Classification of Muscles

Morphological Classification (Based on structure)

1. **Striated**
   - Skeletal muscle
   - Cardiac muscle (Fig. 3.4)
2. **Nonstriated or smooth**
   - Smooth muscle

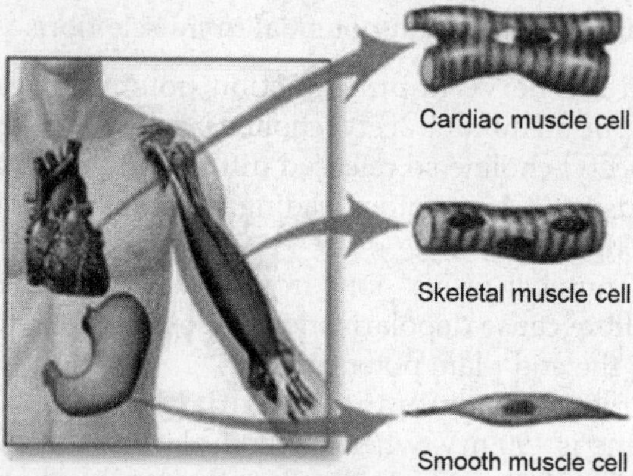

Fig. 3.4: Cardiac muscle

Functional Classification

1. Voluntary
   Skeletal muscle
2. Involuntary
   - Cardiac muscle
   - Smooth muscle

1. **Skeletal—attaches bone to muscle**
   - striated—has cross band(alteration of dark and light cross band).
   - Voluntary—under the will.
   - Multinucleated—cylindrical cell, peripherally located nuclei.

2. **Visceral—smooth muscle**
   - Nonstriated—absent cross band.
   - Involuntary.
   - Uni/binucleated—spindle shape, overlapping sheet with one centrally located oval nucleus.
3. **Cardiac-muscular wall of heart**
   - Striated.
   - Involuntary.
   - Uni/binucleated.

Structure of Skeletal Muscle (Fig. 3.5)

The Muscle Fibre

Skeletal muscle is made up of thousands of cylindrical muscle **fibres** running all the way from origin to insertion. The fibres are bound together by connective tissue through which run blood vessels and nerves.

Each muscle fiber (1–4 cm) long, cylindrical surrounded by a cell membrane called sarcolemma. The cytoplasm in the muscle fibre called sarcoplasm contains:

- Mitochondria.
- An extensive smooth endoplasmic reticulum **(sarcoplasmic reticulum)**.

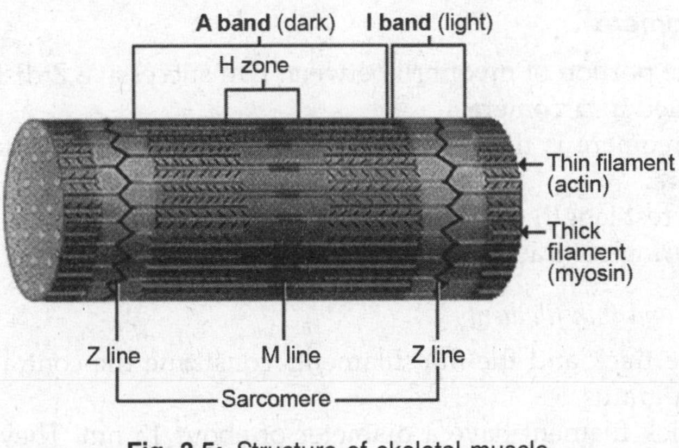

Fig. 3.5: Structure of skeletal muscle

- Many nuclei.
- Ribosomes, glycogen, lipid droplets.

The sarcolemma with sarcoplasmic reticulum is known as **sarcotubular system**.

Each muscle fibre is made up of myofibrils which run parallel to each other.

Myofibril is made up of myofilaments (thick and thin)

The thick filaments consists of **myosin** and the thin filaments consists of **actin**. Skeletal muscle fibers show a peculiar arrangement of these myofilaments which gives rise to alternate light and dark bands (striations) on light microscopy.

Striations of Muscle Fibres

The striated appearance of the muscle fiber is created by a pattern of alternating:

- Dark **A band. It is 1.5 μm in length. In the area of A band thin and thick filaments overlap each other.**
- Light **I band. It is 1 μm in length. It contains only thin filaments.**
- The A bands are bisected by the **H zone** running through the center of which is the **M line**. H zone is that portion of A band where thin and thick filaments do not overlap each other.
- The I bands are bisected by the **Z disc**.

Sarcomere

- The portion of myofibril between two successive Z disks is called a **sarcomere.**
- Sarcomere is the structural and functional unit of muscle fibre.
- At rest length of sarcomere is 2.5 μm
- During contraction length of sarcomere is 1.5 μm (Fig. 3.6).

Thick and thin filaments

- The thick and the thin filaments constitute the contractile apparatus.
- Thick filament have a diameter of about 15 nm. They are composed of protein myosin.

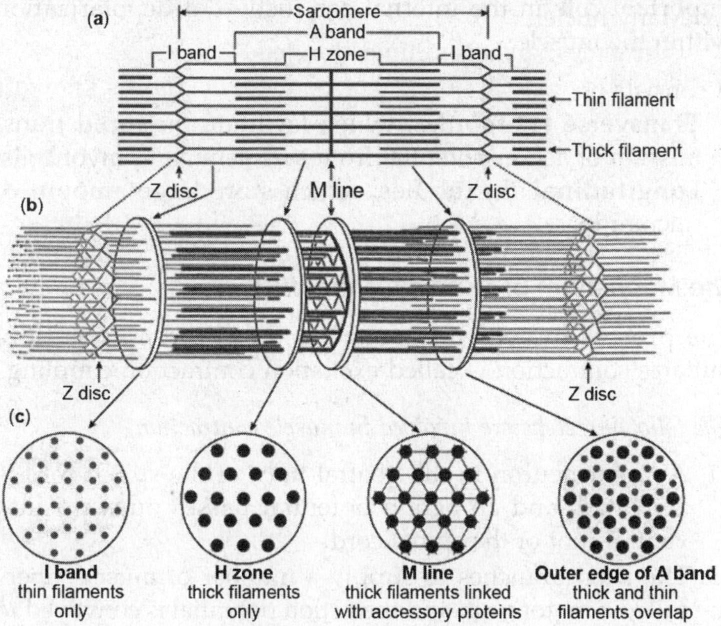

Fig. 3.6: Sarcomere

- Thin filaments have a diameter of about 5 nm.They are composed chiefly of the protein actin along with two smaller proteins:
  - Troponin
  - Tropomyosin (Fig. 3.7).

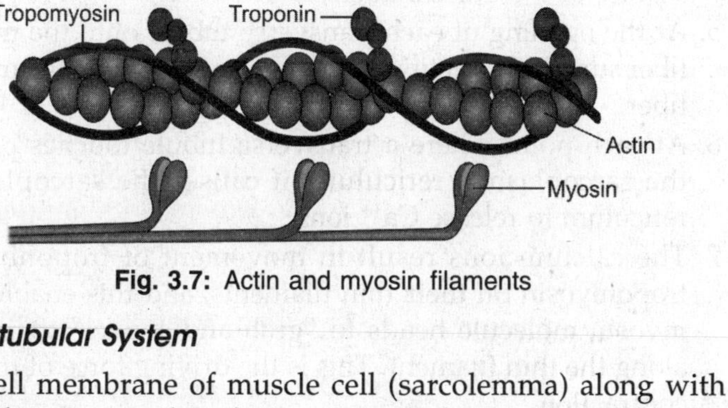

Fig. 3.7: Actin and myosin filaments

Sarcotubular System

The cell membrane of muscle cell (sarcolemma) along with sarcoplasmic reticulum forms sarcotubular system. It plays an important role in the internal conduction of depolarization within the muscle.

It consists of:

- **Transverse** (T) tubules, which facilitate the rapid transmission of action potential from sarcolemma to myofibrils.
- **Longitudinal** (L) tubules, which store large amount of calcium ions.

The Mechanism of Muscle Contraction

The process by which depolarization of the muscle fibre initiates contraction is called excitation contraction coupling.

The following steps are involved in muscle contraction

1. A motor neuron in the ventral horn of the spinal cord is activated, and an action potential passes outward in a ventral root of the spinal cord.
2. The axon branches to supply a number of muscle fibers called a motor unit, and the action potential is conveyed to a motor end plate on each muscle fiber.
3. At the motor end plate, the action potential causes the release of packets or quanta of **acetylcholine** into the **synaptic clefts** on the surface of the muscle fiber.
4. Acetylcholine causes the electrical **resting potential** under the motor end plate to change, and this then initiates an action potential which passes in both directions along the surface of the muscle fiber.
5. At the opening of each transverse tubule onto the muscle fiber surface, the action potential spreads inside the muscle fiber.
6. At each point where a transverse tubule touches part of the sarcoplasmic reticulum, it causes the sarcoplasmic reticulum to release Ca^{++} ions.
7. The calcium ions result in movement of troponin and tropomyosin on their thin filaments, and this enables the myosin molecule heads to "grab and swivel" their way along the thin filament. This is the driving force of muscle contraction.

Contraction is turned off by the following sequence of events

8. Acetylcholine at the neuromuscular junction is broken down by acetylcholinesterase, and this terminates the stream of action potentials along the muscle fiber surface.
9. The sarcoplasmic reticulum ceases to release calcium ions, and immediately starts to resequester all the calcium ions that have been released.
10. In the absence of calcium ions, a change in the configuration of troponin and tropomyosin then blocks the action of the myosin molecule heads, and contraction ceases.

Muscle Contraction (Fig. 3.8)

Contraction Phase

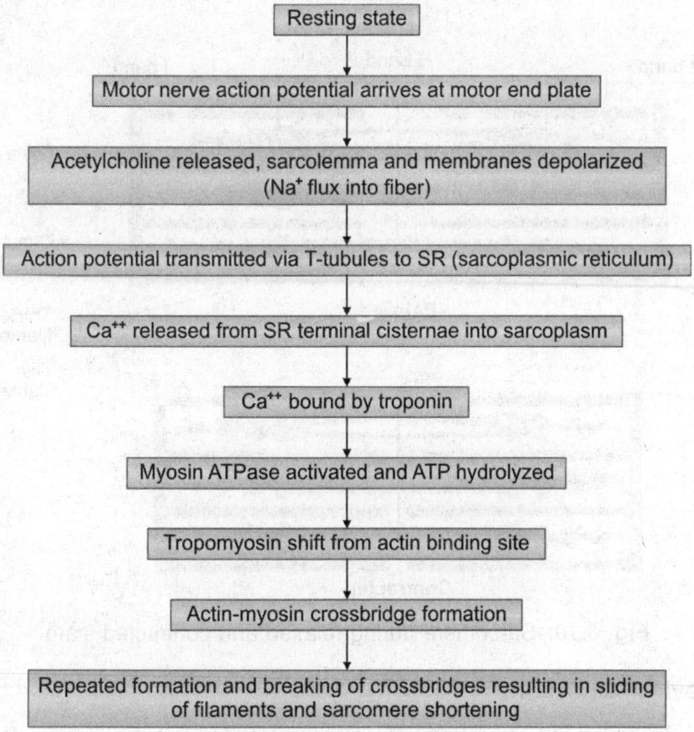

Fig. 3.8: Muscle contraction

Relaxation Phase (Fig. 3.9)

Cholinesterase released and acetylcholine breakdown

↓

Sarcolemma and T-tubules repolarized

↓

SR Ca^{++} pump activated & Ca^{++} returned to SR terminal cisternae

↓

Actin-myosin crossbridge formation terminated

↓

Return of tropomyosin to actin binding site

↓

Sarcomere return to resting state

Fig. 3.9: Muscle relaxation phase

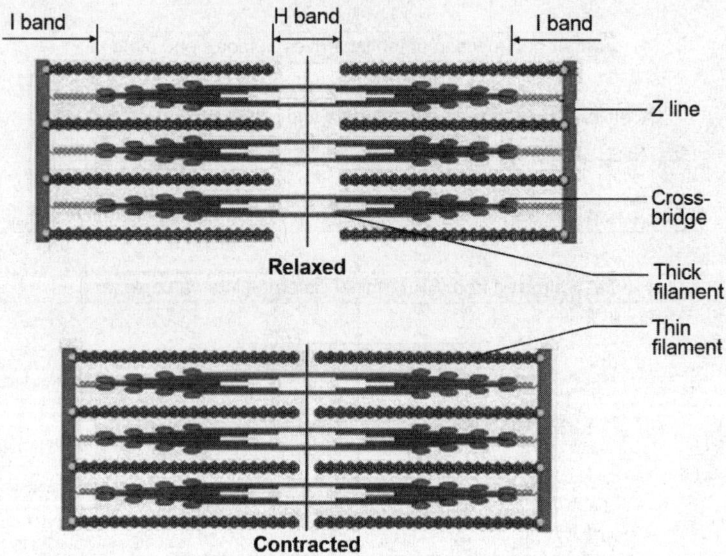

Fig. 3.10: Sarcomere during relaxed and contracted state

Review Questions

1. Describe the structure of neuromuscular junction.
2. Explain neuromuscular transmission.

3. Sketch the diagram for neuromuscular junction with proper labeling.
4. Describe the mechanism of contraction in skeleton muscle
5. Write short notes on:
   - Sarcomere.
   - Sarcotubular system.
   - Classification of muscles.

4 Respiratory System

RESPIRATORY SYSTEM

Pathway of air: nasal cavities (or oral cavity) > pharynx > trachea > primary bronchi (right and left) > secondary bronchi > tertiary bronchi > bronchioles > alveoli (site of gas exchange) (Fig. 4.1).

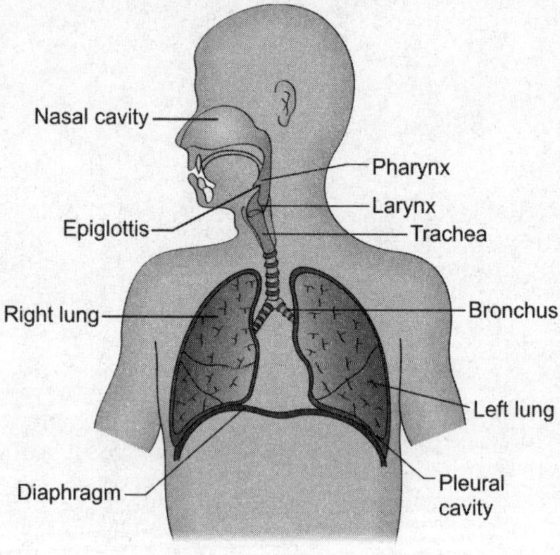

Fig. 4.1: Respiratory system

Functions of Respiratory System

- Transfer of O_2 from the alveoli to the venous blood and CO_2 in the opposite direction.
- Maintenance of pH of the body fluids.
- Regulation of PCO_2 of blood.
- Excretion of certain volatile gases, e.g. chloroform, ether.

Table 4.1: Functional divisions of lungs

Functional organization of the respiratory system	The respiratory system is composed of a network of passageways which permit air to flow from the external environment to the lungs
Nasal cavity	The nasal cavity is exposed to the air through the nostrils which is lined with a ciliated mucous membrane which filters, warms, and moistens the air.
Pharynx	The pharynx is the area in which the oral cavity and nasal cavity meet. Food is prevented from entering the trachea by the epiglottis.
Trachea	The trachea is kept open by rings of cartilage. The ciliated mucous membrane which lines the trachea traps microscopic particles and sweeps them toward the bronchi. Deposits from cigarette smoke and other atmospheric pollutants may interfere with the action of cilia.
Bronchi	The 2 major subdivisions of the trachea are the bronchi. The bronchi are lined with mucous membrane and ringed with cartilage. Each bronchus extends into a lung where it subdivides many times forming progressively smaller bronchioles.
Bronchioles	Bronchioles are lined with mucous membrane but lack cartilage rings and no cilia present. Tiny bronchioles terminate with the alveoli.
Alveoli	Alveoli are the functional units for gas exchange. They are thin, moist, and surrounded by capillaries. In humans, oxyhemoglobin is in highest concentration in the capillaries of alveoli.
Lung	Each bronchus with its bronchioles and alveoli is called a lung.

- Respiratory muscles are used during laughing, singing.
- Metabolic functions of lungs are:
  1. Formation of surfactant.
  2. Secretion of immunoglobulins (IgA).

MECHANICS OF RESPIRATION

Eupnoea means rhythmic breathing at rest. It consists of inspiration and expiration (Table 4.2).

Table 4.2: Mechanism of respiration

Inhalation (inspiration) active phase	1. Diaphragm pulled down 2. Ribs pulled up and out 3. (–) pressure causes air to fill lungs
Exhalation (expiration) passive phase	1. Diaphragm relaxes, comes up 2. Ribs relax, drop down and in 3. (+) pressure forces air out of lungs

Inspiration

1. It is an active process.
2. Expansion of the lungs during inspiration follows the enlargement of the thoracic cavity in all its diameter by contraction of the respiratory muscles.
3. Inspiration commences by contraction of the diaphragm increasing the vertical diameter of the thoracic cage.
4. Movement of ribs outwards and upwards due to contraction of external intercostals muscles increasing the antero-posterior and transverse diameter of the chest.

Mechanism of Expiration

It is passive process which occurs due to relaxation of inspiratory muscles.

Pressure changes during ventilation

1. ***Intra pulmonary pressure:*** It is the pressure within the lung parenchyma.
   Normally, at the end of inspiration and expiration, the intra pulmonary pressure is equal to atmospheric pressure (760 mm Hg).
   With inspiration it decreases by 3 mm Hg, i.e. 757 mm Hg) while with expiration it increases by 3 mm Hg, i.e. 763 mm Hg).
2. ***Intra pleural pressure:*** It is the pressure between 2 layers of pleura. The intra pleural pressure is slightly negative during resting stage (–2 mm of Hg) and becomes more negative to –6 mm Hg during inspiration.

TRANSPORT OF GASES

O_2 Transport

O_2 is transported through blood in two forms.
1. Dissolved in plasma (3%).
2. In combination with hemoglobin (97%).

Dissolved State

Oxygen dissolves in water of the plasma and is transported in this physical form. It is only 0.3 mL/100 ml of plasma, i.e. 3%. This form of transport is important in conditions like exercise.

In combination with haemoglobin: Haemoglobin combines with O_2 reversibly to form oxyhaemoglobin. When O_2 is released from Hb, it is termed as reduced haemoglobin (Fig. 4.2).

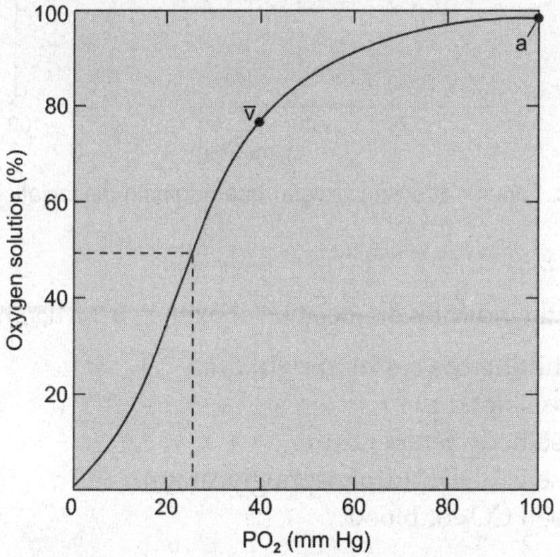

Fig. 4.2: Oxygen hemoglobin dissociation curve

- 1 gm of Hb combines with 1.34 ml of O_2.
- Oxygen Hb dissociation curve relates % O_2 saturation of Hb to PO_2 (partial pressure of O_2).
- It has a characteristic sigmoid shape. The lower part of the curve indicates dissociation of oxygen from haemoglobin and the upper indicates acceptance of oxygen by haemoglobin.

Factors affecting oxygen haemoglobin dissociation curve

The oxygen haemoglobin dissociation curve is shifted to right or left by various factors (Fig. 4.3).

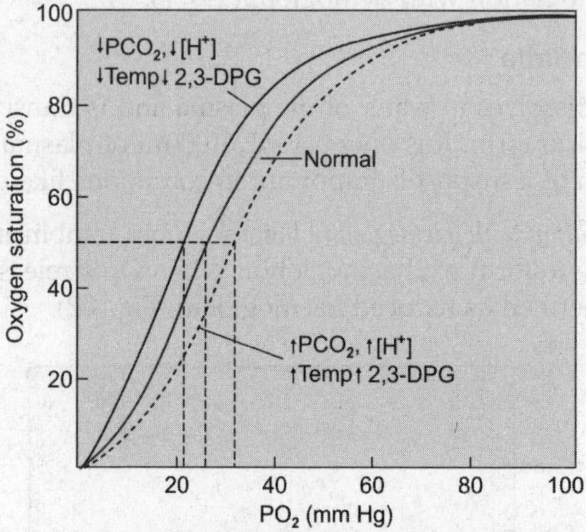

Fig. 4.3: Factors affecting oxygen haemoglobin dissociation curve

Shift to right

Shift to right indicates dissociation of oxygen from haemoglobin.

Factors shifting the curve to right are:

- Decrease blood pH
- Increase body temperature.
- Increase 2,3-DPG (diphosphoglycerate).
- Increase PCO_2 of blood.

Shift to left

Shift to left indicates acceptance of oxygen by haemoglobin.

Factors shifting the curve to left are:

- Decrease PCO_2 of blood.
- Increase pH of blood.
- Decrease temperature.
- Fetal haemoglobin.

Transport of CO_2

Carbon dioxide is transported by the blood from tissues to the alveoli. Carbon dioxide is transported by the following mechanisms:

1. ***Dissolved state in plasma (70%):*** Carbon dioxide dissolves in the fluid of plasma. In this form only about 3 ml/100 ml of CO_2 is transported.
2. ***In bicarbonate form (7%):*** After entering the blood CO_2 combines with water to form carbonic acid (H_2CO_3) which dissociates into H^+ and HCO_3^- ions. This reaction occurs in the RBCs at a very high rate due to enzyme carbonic anhydrase. H^+ ions are buffered by haemoglobin and HCO_3^- passes out from cell to plasma.
3. ***In carbaminocompound from (23%):*** CO_2 reacts directly with amino group of the proteins, haemoglobin and plasma proteins to form carbaminocompounds.

REGULATION OF RESPIRATION

Regulation of respiration is by two mechanisms
1. Nervous/neural
2. Chemical.

Nervous Mechanism

Respiratory Centres

Respiratory centres are group of neurons which controls the rate, rhythm and force of respiration. They are situated in the brainstem (Fig. 4.4).

The respiratory centres are classified into two groups:

Medullary Centres

- Dorsal respiratory groups of neurons
- Ventral respiratory groups of neurons

Pontine Centres

1. Pneumotaxic
2. Apneustic

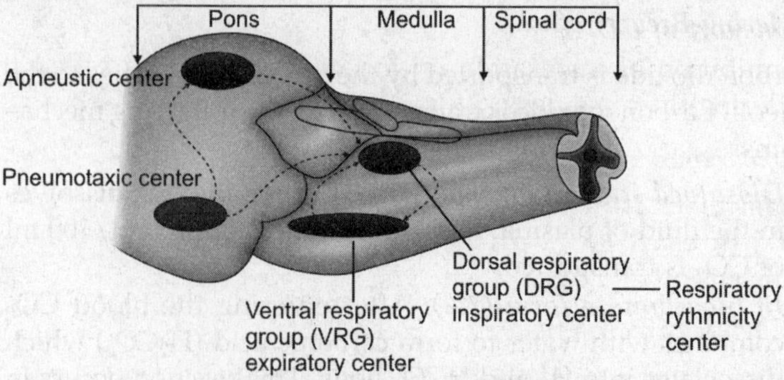

Fig. 4.4: Respiratory centres

Dorsal respiratory groups of neurons: Dorsal respiratory group of neurons are diffusely situated in the nucleus of tractus solitarus in the upper part of medulla oblongata.

Functions

They are responsible for the basic rhythm of respiration.

Ventral respiratory group of neurons: These neurons are present in nucleus ambiguous and nucleus retroambiguous.

Function

The ventral group of neurons are inactive during quiet breathing but becomes active during forced breathing. Whenever there is increased pulmonary ventilation, this area contributes to both inspiration and expiration, provides strong signals to expiratory muscles.

Pneumotaxic centre: It is present in the upper pons.

Function

The primary function of this centre is to control the duration of inspiration.

Apneustic centre: It is present in the lower pons

Function

This centre operates in association with pneumotaxic centre to control depth of inspiration.

Hering-Breuer reflex

Inhibition of inspiration on inflation of lungs is called the Hering-Breuer reflex.

Importance

This reflex is initiated only when the tidal volume is more than 1.5 litres. It has a protective role in preventing excessive distension of lungs.

Chemical mechanism

The chemical regulation of respiration is by the help of chemo receptors. These receptors sense the chemical changes in blood.

They are classified into two groups:

1. ***Central chemoreceptors:*** They are situated in the medulla close to the dorsal respiratory group of neurons.
2. ***Peripheral chemoreceptors:*** They are situated in the aortic and carotid bodies.

Chemoreceptors are stimulated by:

- Hypoxia (decreased PO_2).
- Hypercapnia (increased CO_2).
- Increased H^+ ions concentration.

HYPOXIA

Hypoxia is defined as reduced availability of oxygen to the tissues.

Types of hypoxia:

1. Hypoxic hypoxia.
2. Stagnant hypoxia.
3. Anaemic hypoxia.
4. Histotoxic hypoxia.

Hypoxic Hypoxia

It means decreased oxygen content of blood.

Causes

- High attitude
- Respiratory disorders like damage to respiratory centre, paralysis of respiratory muscles like poliomyelitis.
- Congenital heart disease.

Stagnant Hypoxia

It is the hypoxia due to inadequate rate of blood flow to the tissues.

Causes

- Congestive cardiac failure.
- Haemorrhage.
- Thrombosis.

Anaemic Hypoxia

It is due to decrease in the oxygen carrying capacity of blood.

Causes

- Decreased numbers of RBCs.
- Decreased haemoglobin.
- Altered haemoglobin.

Histotoxic Hypoxia

Decreased ability of tissues to utilize oxygen is called histotoxic hypoxia

Causes

Cyanide poisoning

ASPHYXIA

Asphyxia is the condition characterized by hypoxia (decreased O_2) and hypercapnoea (increased CO_2).

Causes

- Strangulation.
- Hanging.
- Drowning.

PULMONARY FUNCTION TEST

Pulmonary function test or lung function tests are useful in assessing the functional status of the respiratory system. They are carried out by using spirometer. The air in the lungs is classified into two divisions (Fig. 4.5).

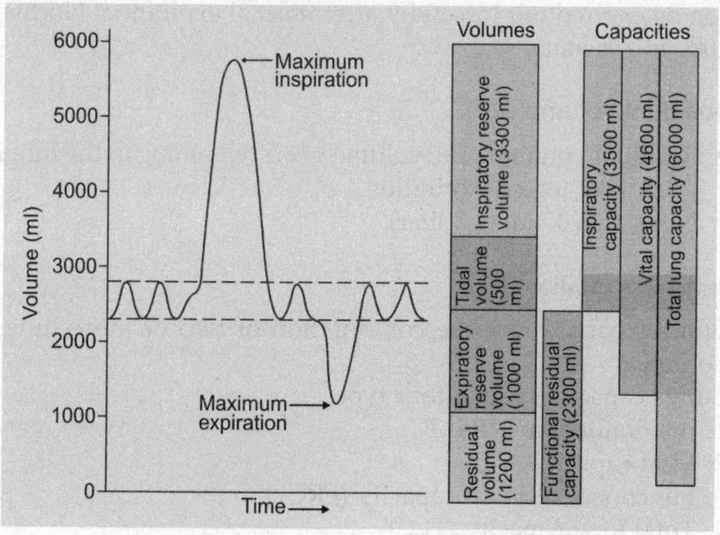

Fig. 4.5: Pulmonary function test

1. Lung volumes.
2. Lung capacities.

Lung Volumes

The lung volumes are of four types:
1. Tidal volume.
2. Inspiratory reserve volume.
3. Expiratory reserve volume.
4. Residual volume.

Tidal Volume (TV)

Tidal volume is the volume of air breathed in and out of lungs in a single normal quite respiration. Normal 500 mL (0.5 liter)

Inspiratory Reserve Volume (IRV)

Inspiratory reserve volume is an additional volume of air that can be inspired forcefully after the end of normal inspiration. Normal 3300 mL (3.3 liters).

Expiratory Reserve Volume (ERV)

Expiratory reserve volume is the additional volume of air that can be expired out forcefully after normal expiration. Normal 1000 mL (1 liter).

Residual Volume (RV)

- Residual volume is the volume of air remaining in the lungs even after forced expiration.
- Normal 1200 ml (1.2 liter).

Lung Capacities (LC)

Lung capacities are the combination of two or more lungs volumes

Lungs capacities are of four types:

1. Inspiratory capacity (IC).
2. Vital capacity (VC).
3. Functional residual capacity (FRC).
4. Total lung capacity (TLC).

Inspiratory Capacity (IC)

- Inspiratory capacity is the maximum volume of air which can be inspired after normal expiration.
- IC = TV + IRV. Normal value: 2500–3700 ml.

Functional Residual Capacity (FRC)

- It is the volume of air which is present in the lungs after completion of tidal expiration. It can be computed as RV+ERV.
- Normal value: 2.5 litres.

Total Lung Capacity (TLC)

- It is the volume of air present in the lungs after a maximal inspiration. It is computed as VC + RV.
- Normal value:6 litres.

Vital Capacity (VC)

- It is the maximal volume of air which can be expelled from the lungs by forceful effort following a maximal inspiration

- Normal value : 4.8 litres in males and 3.2 litres in females.
- It can be computed as : TV + IRV + ERV.

Advantages of VC

It provides useful information about the strength of the respiratory muscles.

Factors Affecting Vital Capacity

Physiological

1. *Age:* vital capacity decreases in old age
2. *Sex*: less in females
3. *Body built:* Vital capacity slightly more in heavy built persons.
4. *Athletes:* Vital capacity more in athletes
5. *Posture:* Vital capacity is more in standing position and less in lying position.

Pathological

Vital capacity is reduced in following respiratory conditions:
1. Asthma
2. Weakness of respiratory muscles
3. Pneumonia.

Forced Vital Capacity

- Forced vital capacity is the volume of air which can be expired forcefully in a given unit of time. It is also called timed vital capacity.
- FEV_1 (forced expiratory volume in 1 sec); it is the volume of FVC expired in 1st sec of exhalation. Normal: 80% of FVC.
- FEV_2 forced expiratory volume in 2 sec); it is the volume of FVC in 1st two sec of exhalation. Normal: 95% of FVC.
- FEV_3 (forced expiratory volume in 3 sec); it is the volume of FVC in 1st three sec of exhalation.
- Normal: 100% of FVC.
- Clinical significant of FVC is to distinguish between restrictive and obstructive lung disorders.
- Restrictive: kyphoscoliosis, polio myelitis.
- Obstructive: asthma, emphysema.

Peak Expiratory Flow Rate

- It is the maximum rate at which air can be expired after a deep inspiration
- Normal: 400 litres/min
- It is reduced in obstructive lung disorders.

Review Questions

1. Enumerate the functions of respiratory system.
2. Describe the transport of gases (O_2 and CO_2).
3. Write in brief about regulation of respiration.
4. Draw a well labeled diagram of lung volumes and capacities.
5. Write in brief the mechanism of respiration.
6. Write short note on:
   a. Pulmonary function test.
   b. Organization of respiratory system.
   c. Hypoxia.
   d. Asphyxia.

5 Cardiovascular System

The cardiovascular system functions can be categorized into three main functions:

1. Transport
2. Regulation
3. Protection

The organs of this system carry out these functions in coordination with the functions of the other systems for the proper functioning of the body, as explained below.

Transport

The cardiovascular system transports oxygen from the lungs to the various cells of the body. The primary function of the cardiovascular system is to transport nutrients from the intestines to the other parts of the body, and carbon dioxide from the cells to the lungs. Hormones from the various endocrine glands and heat from the cells are also transported by this system. Removal of waste products like carbon dioxide and nitrogen from the body is also performed by this system.

Protection

The CVS performs the function of protecting the body from infections by providing the white blood cells and antibodies required for destroying viruses, bacteria, etc.

Regulation

Another important cardiovascular system function is the regulation of the concentration of hydrogen ions (pH) in the body, the body temperature and body heat, and the regulation of the salt and water content of the cells in the body.

CARDIOVASCULAR SYSTEM FUNCTION AND STRUCTURE

The cardiovascular system is made up of the heart and the blood vessels.

The Heart

The human heart is situated at the center of the chest and is approximately the size of a clenched fist. It performs the function of a muscular pump, wherein it expands and contracts to pump blood into the blood vessels and the body. The deoxygenated blood is carried to the right side of the heart which pumps it into the lungs where blood absorbs more oxygen. This oxygenated blood moves to the left side of the heart which pumps it into the blood stream and is carried to the various body parts.

Blood Vessels

There are three different types of blood vessels in the human body the arteries, the capillaries and the veins. The arteries are of three types, the pulmonary artery, the aorta and the coronary arteries. They perform the function of carrying oxygenated blood from the heart to the other parts of the body, but the pulmonary artery carries deoxygenated blood from the heart to the lungs. The capillaries carry oxygen and nutrients to the tissues and cells of the body and the veins carry deoxygenated blood from the various organs of the body to the heart.

Organization

The human heart weighs approximately 300 gm and contains 4 chambers.

- Two thin walled atria separated from each other by an inter atrial septum.
- Two thick walled ventricles separated from each other by an interventricular septum.

Valves in the Heart

A. *Atrio ventricular valves (AV valves):* Tricuspid and mitral valves.

B. *Semilunar valves:* Pulmonary and aortic valves.

- Pulmonary valve is situated at pulmonary orifice which leads from the right ventricle (RV) to the pulmonary artery.
- Aortic valve is situated at the aortic orifice which lead from the left ventricle (LV) to the aorta.

Function

The valves prevent the regurgitation of blood into the atria but allows it to flow out of the ventricles. In this way circulation becomes one way.

Pacemaker Tissue of the Heart

Definition

Tissues in the heart concerned with the generation and conduction of the heartbeat.

These include the following

- Sinoatrial node (SAN).
- Atrioventricular node (AVN).
- Atrioventricular bundle (bundle of His).
- Purkinje fibers.

Conduction speed in cardiac tissue:

Cardiac tissue	Conduction speed (m/s)
SAN	0.05
AV Node	0.05
Bundle of His	1.0
Purkinje system	4.0 (fastest)

Sinus node, it is situated in the right atrium and generates the normal rhythmical cardiac impulse at the rate of 70–80 beats per minute and acts as a pacemaker of heart. The rhythm generated from this region in called sinus rhythm.

Internodal pathways conduct the impulse from the sinus node to the AV node.

AV node receives the impulse originating from the SA node and transmits it to the ventricles through the Bundle of His. In abnormal conditions when the SA node fails to generate impulse, it can also initiate the cardiac impulse but at a slower rate (40–60 per minute).

The AV Bundle conducts the impulse from the atria to the ventricles.

The right and left bundle branches conduct the cardiac impulse to the ventricles.

Purkinje fibres, the main function of these fibres is to conduct impulse quickly to every part of the ventricular muscle fibres.

Cardiac Cycle

Definition

- The sequence of changes in the pressure and blood flow in the heart chambers and blood vessels from beat to beat is called cardiac cycle (Fig. 5.1).
- Normal duration: 0.8 sec

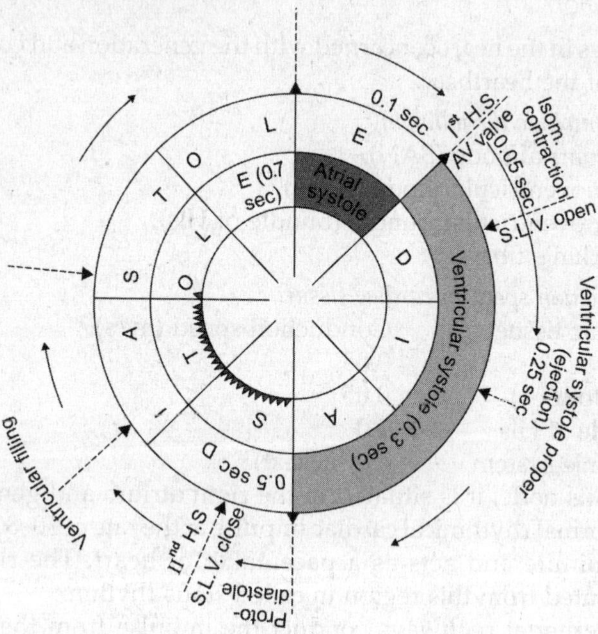

Fig. 5.1: Cardiac cycle

Events:

- Atrial systole: 0.1 sec.
- Atrial diastole: 0.7 sec.
- Ventricular systole: 0.3 sec.
- Ventricular diastole: 0.5 sec.

Atrial systole (0.1 sec)

Atrial systole initiates the cardiac cycle. During this period the atria contract and expel their contents into the ventricles.

Atrial diastole (0.7 sec)

During this period the atria relax receives blood from the great veins. The right atrium from the superior and inferior venae cavae and the coronary sinus. The left atrium from the pulmonary veins.

Ventricular systole (0.3 sec)

It has two major phases:
1. Isovolumetric ventricular contraction (0.05 sec.)
2. Ventricular systole proper (0.25 sec).

Isovolumetric ventricular contraction:

During this period ventricular contraction begins and ventricular pressure exceeds atrial pressure causing closure of the AV valves with production of first heart sound. Although contraction is occurring in the ventricles but there is no emptying.

Ventricular systole proper

- It is associated with ejection of blood out of the ventricles.
- When the pressure is the LV exceeds the pressure in the aorta (80 mm Hg) and pressure in the RV exceeds the pressure in the pulmonary artery (10–12) mm Hg opening of semi lunar valves occurs (aortic and pulmonary). With opening of semi lunar valves, there is ejection of blood from the ventricles.
- The amount of blood ejected by each ventricle per stroke is 70–80 ml. This is called stroke volume.

Ventricular diastole (0.5 sec)

- Protodiastole.
- Ventricular diastole proper.

Protodiastole

At the end of ventricular systole, the intra ventricular pressure drops and the atrial pressure exceed that in the ventricles. This result in closure of semi lunar valves causing sharp production of second heart sound.

Ventricular diastole

During this phase atrial blood rushes into the ventricles and ventricular filling occurs.

Heart Sounds

There are two classical sounds of the heart, known as the first and the second sounds which can be easily detected with a stethoscope, the two other sounds third and fourth have also been described, are difficult to detect clinically but can be recorded graphically (phonocardiogram).

First heart sound

It occurs at the onset of ventricular systole.

Cause

It is due to closure of AV valves

Character

- Low pitch
- Loud
- Sound like syllable L-U-B-B.
  Duration: 0.1–0.17 sec

Site

It can be heard all over the chest but best heard over mitral and tricuspid areas.

Second heart sound

It occurs at the onset of diastole.

Cause

It is due to the closure of semilunar valves

Character

- High pitch
- Sharp
- Second like the syllable D-U-P-P.
- Duration: 0.1–0.14 sec.

Site

It can be heard all are over chest but best heard over pulmonary and aortic areas.

Blood Pressure

The arterial blood pressure (BP) is the lateral pressure exerted by the column of blood in the arterial system

Factors Affecting BP

Age

Blood pressure rises with age.

Sex

In females less by 4–5 mm Hg, up to the age of 45–50 years (oestrogen effect).

Body built

The systolic pressure is usually more in obese people.

Diurnal variation

Common with SBP (peak during afternoon and lowest during early hours of morning)

Exercise

- In untrained individuals there is increase in systolic BP in mild, moderate and severe exercise. Diastolic BP is increased in moderate to severe exercises.
- Whereas in trained individuals no effect on BP in moderate exercise with slight increase in systolic BP with severe exercises.

Emotions

Excitement, fear causes rise in systolic blood pressure.

Sleep

The systolic pressure falls by 15–20 mm of Hg during sleep.

Posture

The diastolic pressure is slightly higher in standing position.

Meals

There is a slight increase in SBP after ingestion of meals.

Components of Blood Pressure (Table 5.1)

Determinants of Blood Pressure *(Factor controlling BP)*

Pumping action of the heart

Effective contraction of the heart is the main factor for controlling cardiac output, blood pressure and blood flow within the blood vessel.

Cardiac output

- BP is a function of **CO X PR**.
  - CO-Cardiac output
  - PR-Peripheral resistance.
- Alterations of cardiac output will alter the blood pressure. Cardiac output depends upon venous return, force and frequency of heart beat.
- As **CO=HR X SV**.
  - HR-Heart rate.
  - SV- Stroke volume.

Therefore alterations in either heart rate or stoke volume will affect blood pressure by modifying cardiac output.

Peripheral Resistance

It is resistance which blood has to overcome while passing through the periphery. Peripheral resistance depends upon the following factors.

- Velocity of blood flow.
- Viscosity of blood flow.
- Total quantity of blood in arterial system.
- Elasticity of the vessel wall.

Regulation of Blood Pressure

The main aim of regulation of BP is to maintain MBP with a normal range of 95–100 mmHg. The mechanism is as follows:

Table 5.1: Components of blood pressure

SR No	*Component*	*Definition*	*Significant features*	*Normal range*
1.	Systolic blood pressure (SBP)	Maximum pressure exerted during systole	Subjected to fluctuations and indicates the extent of work done by heart	Range 100–130 mm Hg Average 120 mm Hg
2.	Diastolic blood pressure (DBP)	Minimum pressure exerted during diastole	It is a measure of total peripheral resistance.	Range 60–80 Average 70 mm Hg
3	Pulse pressure (PP)	PP=SBP-DBP	Determines the pulse volume and varies directly as stroke volume.	Average 50 mm Hg
4	Mean blood pressure (MBP)	It the average pressure throughout the cardiac cycle given as MBP = DBP + 1/3PP	Determines the pressure head for blood flow through an organ.	Range 90–100 mm Hg

A. ***Rapid acting regulatory mechanism***

This includes:
- Baroreceptor reflexes.
- Chemoreceptor reflexes.
- CNS ischaemic reflexes.

B. ***Intermediate acting regulatory mechanism***

This includes:
- Capillary fluid shift mechanism.
- Stress relaxation mechanism.

C. ***Long-term regulatory mechanism:*** This is mainly done by kidneys either by controlling blood volume or by hormonal system (aldosterone and renin-angiotensin mechanisms).

Cardiac Output

Definition

- The amount of blood pumped out by each ventricle per minute is called cardiac output. The output of the two ventricles is exactly the same.
- Normally it is 5–6 litres/min.

Distribution of cardiac output

- 25% liver.
- 25% kidney.
- 25% brain, heart, lung.
- 25% skin, skeletal muscle and other body organs.
- Cardiac index.

The cardiac output per minute per square meter of body surface is known as cardiac index. It is 3.3 litres/min/m^2.

Factors Influencing Cardiac Output

Muscular exercise: In heavy exercise cardiac output may increase to 30–40 litres.

Fever, hyperthyroidism, excitement, adrenaline, ingestion of food increase cardiac output.

Hypothyroidism, haemorrhage, shock, reduce cardiac output.

Sleep: May slightly reduce cardiac output.

Control of cardiac output (regulation)

As CO = HR × SV, therefore cardiac output is controlled by two main mechanisms:

1. Control of HR (heart rate)
2. Control of SV (stroke volume).

A. Control of heart rate

Normal resting HR in adult is 70–80 beats/min

Factors affecting heart rate

Age: As age increases heart rate decreases

Sex: Slightly higher in females.

Body temperature: HR increases with increase in body temperature.

Emotional stimuli increases HR

Exercise increases HR.

Heart rate regulation depends mainly upon:

- cardiac innervations (sympathetic and parasympathetic nerve supply).
- Medullary cardiovascular centres.

B. Stroke volume

Stroke volume depends upon:

- The end diastolic volume which in turn is affected by venous return.
- Myocardial contractility.

Venous Return

Increase in the venous return, increases the end-diastolic volume which in turn increases the force of myocardial contraction and stoke volume.

Factors affecting venous return

1. ***Respiratory pump:*** There is increase in venous return during inspiration
2. ***Cardiac pump:*** Blood in the veins is attracted towards the heart by contraction of the ventricles.

3. ***Blood volume:*** Increase in blood volume increases venous return.
4. ***Muscle pump:*** Contraction of skeletal muscle squeezes the veins of the lower limbs and propels the bloods towards heart.
5. ***Body position:*** In standing posture there is peripheral pooling of the blood and decrease in venous return.

Myocardial contractility

It is increased by:

- Sympathetic stimulation.
- Drugs like digitalis.

Decreased by:

- Stimulation of vagus.
- Heart failure.
- Myocardial infarction.

Method of measurement of cardiac output

Cardiac output can be determined by the following methods:

- Fick's principle
- Indicator (dye) dilution method
- Echocardiography

Shock

Definition

It is defined as generalized inadequacy of blood to flow throughout the body, to the extent that body tissues get damaged due to too little delivery of O_2 and nutrients.

Classification

- Hypovolemic shock (haemorrhagic).
- Vasogenic shock.
- Cardiogenic shock.
- Obstructive shock.

Haemorrhagic/Hypovolemic

It is due to decrease in circulating blood volume, e.g. external or internal haemorrhage (injury, fracture) fluid loss—diarrhea, vomiting, burns.

Vasogenic shock

- It is due to decrease in the vascular tone of venous reservoirs
- Emotional fainting
- Anaphylaxis (due to allergic reaction)
- Sepsis (blood borne infection) like peritonitis.

Cardiogenic shock

It is due to decrease in the pumping ability of the heart because of cardiac abnormalities, e.g. myocardial infarction, heart valve dysfunction, congestive heart failure.

Obstructive shock

It is due to obstruction of blood flow in heart or lungs, e.g. pulmonary embolism, cardiac tumor.

Sign and symptoms

1. Decreased blood pressure.
2. Tachycardia.
3. Pale and cold skin.
4. Rapid respiration.
5. Agitation, restlessness.

Stages of shock

- ***Non progressive:*** Normal circulatory compensatory mechanism leading to full recovery without help of external therapy.
- ***Progressive stage:*** Shock becomes worse until death.
- ***Irreversible stage:*** Shock progresses to such an extent that even therapy is inadequate to save the life of the person.

Compensatory mechanism occurring in shock include

1. Baroreceptor reflex.
2. Chemoreceptor reflex.
3. CNS ischemic response.
4. Reverse stress relaxation.
5. Release of plasma volume by kidneys.
6. Restoration of RBC by increase in erythropoietin.
7. Restoration of plasma proteins by liver.

Treatment

- Fluid replacement–dextran, blood.
- Sympathomimetic drugs.
- O_2 therapy
- Steroids

Review Questions

1. Describe cardiac cycle.
2. Define blood pressure. Enumerate the different types of blood pressure.
3. What is cardiac output? What are the factors affecting cardiac output?
4. Classify shock.
5. Write short notes on:
   - Heart sounds.
   - Functions of cardiovascular system.
   - Regulation of blood pressure.

6 Digestive System

ORGANIZATION AND FUNCTIONS OF GASTROINTESTINAL TRACT (Fig. 6.1)

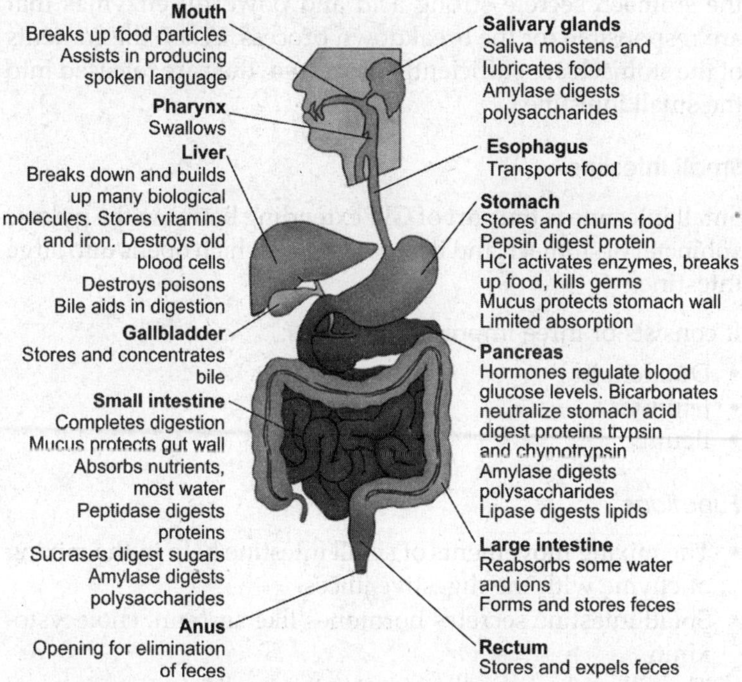

Fig. 6.1: Functions of various parts of gastrointestinal tract

Mouth

The mouth is the beginning of the digestive tract; and, in fact, digestion starts here when taking the first bite of food. Chewing breaks the food into pieces that are more easily digested, while saliva mixes with food to begin the process of breaking it down into a form the body can absorb and use.

Oesophagus

Oesophagus receives food from mouth and by a series of muscular contractions called peristalsis; the esophagus delivers food to stomach.

Stomach

The stomach is a hollow organ, or "container," that holds food while it is being mixed with enzymes that continue the process of breaking down food into a usable form. Cells in the lining of the stomach secrete strong acid and powerful enzymes that are responsible for the breakdown process. When the contents of the stomach are sufficiently processed, they are released into the small intestine.

Small Intestine

Small intestine is the part of GIT extending between the pyloric sphincter of stomach and ileocecal valve, which opens into large intestine.

It consists of three important portions:

- Duodenum.
- Jejunum.
- Ileum.

Functions

- The mixing movements of small intestine help in the mixing of chyme with the digestive juices.
- Small intestine secretes hormones like secretin, cholecysto-kinin.
- The villi and microvilli present in the small intestine, increase the surface area for absorption. The digested products of carbohydrates, proteins, fats and other substances like vitamins, minerals are easily absorbed in the small intestine.
- Enzymes (peptidase, lipase) present in the small intestine helps in the digestion of food.
- Small intestine helps in the absorption of vitamin B_{12}, required for erythropoiesis .

Pancreas

The pancreas secretes digestive enzymes into the duodenum, the first segment of the small intestine. These enzymes break down protein, fats, and carbohydrates. The pancreas also makes insulin, secreting it directly into the bloodstream. Insulin is the chief hormone for metabolizing sugar.

Gallbladder

The gallbladder stores and concentrates bile, and then releases it into the duodenum to help absorb and digest fats.

Liver

Liver is the largest gland in the body weighing 1.5 kg. It performs many vital metabolic and hormonal functions.

Functions of liver are summarized as below:

- ***Metabolic function:*** Liver plays an important role in metabolism of proteins, carbohydrates, fats, vitamins and many hormones.
- ***Secretion of bile:*** Bile secreted by liver helps in breakdown of fats and carry away waste products which are finally excreted through feces or urine.
- ***Excretory function:*** Liver excretes cholesterol, bile pigments, heavily metals, bacteria, etc. through bile.
- ***Hemopoietic function:*** In fetal life, liver produces blood cells. It also stores necessary vitamins and iron required for synthesis of haemoglobin.
- ***Hemolytic function:*** The senile RBCs are destroyed in the liver.
- ***Defense and detoxification function***
  - Liver is involved in the detoxification of harmful substances.
  - The reticuloendothelial cells of liver helps in the phagocytosis of bacterial and other antigens.
- ***Storage function:*** Liver is an important storage organ for vitamins, amino acids, glycogen.
- ***Synthetic function:*** Liver produces glucose, plasma proteins, clotting factors, heparin, etc.

Large Intestine

The large intestine is also known as colon.

It consists of seven parts:
1. Cecum with appendix.
2. Ascending colon.
3. Transverse colon.
4. Descending colon.
5. Sigmoid colon.
6. Rectum.
7. Anal canal.

Functions of Large Intestine

- Large intestine plays an important role in the absorption of water, electrolytes, glucose, alcohol and certain drugs.
- It forms and stores feces until it is expelled out.
- Large intestine secretes mucin, which helps in lubrication and protection of mucous membrane of large intestine by mechanical and chemical injury.
- The bacterial flora of large intestine synthesize folic acid, vitamin B_{12} and vitamin K.

Rectum

The rectum (latin for "straight") is an 8-inch chamber that connects the colon to the anus. It receives stool from the colon, and hold the stool until evacuation happens. When anything (gas or stool) comes into the rectum, sensors send a message to the brain. The brain then decides if the rectal contents can be released or not. If they can, the sphincters relax and the rectum contracts, disposing its contents.

Anus

The anus is the last part of the digestive tract. It is a 2-inch long canal consisting of the pelvic floor muscles and the two anal sphincters (internal and external). The anus is surrounded by sphincter muscles that are important in allowing control of stool.

Defecation

Process by which fecal matter is excreted is called defecation.

Mass peristalsis or mass movements propels the feces into sigmoid colon. The rectum is usually empty, desire for defecation occurs when some feces enters the rectum due to mass movements and initiates defecation reflex. The process of defecation involves contraction of rectum and relaxation of internal and external anal sphincter.

Defecation reflex involves

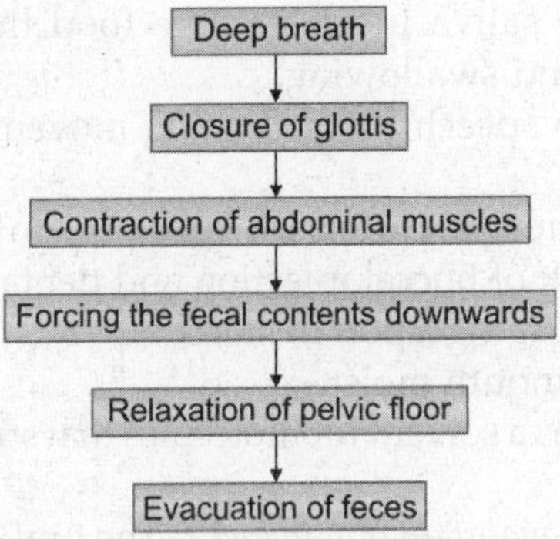

Secretory Functions of GIT

Salivary Glands

Salivary glands includes:

1. Parotid gland.
2. Submandibular gland.
3. Sublingual gland.
4. Buccal gland.

Saliva

Composition

Daily secretion: 1500 mL/day.

Digestive enzymes:

- Ptyalin
- Lingual lipase
- Lysozymes

- Mucin
- Immunoglobulins-IgA

Cations

Na^+ – 15 mEq/L
K^+ – 30 mEq/L
Cl^- – 15 mEq/L
HCO_3^- – 10–15 mEq/L
pH – 6.0–7.0

Functions of Saliva

- Mucin in the saliva lubricates the food thus assisting in mastication and swallowing.
- It also aids in speech by facilitating movements of lip and tongue.
- The lysozymes, lactoferrin, IgA present in the saliva minimizes risk of buccal infection and dental caries.
- Ptyalin helps in digestion of starch.
- Saliva keeps mouth moist.
- Saliva serves as a solvent for molecules that stimulate the taste buds.
- *Saliva helps in maintain oral hygiene:* The oral cavity is almost constantly flushed with saliva, which floats away food debris and keeps the mouth relatively clean.

Gastric Juice

Composition

- Daily secretion: 2500–3000 mL/day
- Electrolytes: Na^+, K^+, Cl^-, H^+, HCO_3^-
- pH: 1–2

Enzymes

- Pepsinogen→pepsin (digestion of proteins)
- Renin (in infants) curdles milk.
- Gastric lipase weak fat splitting enzyme.
- Lysozymes—bactericidal
- Urease—hydrolyse urea to ammonia.
- Mucus: protective and lubricating function.
- Intrinsic factor required for absorption of vitamin B_{12}.
- Water.

Phases of secretion of gastric juice

- Cephalic phase.
- Gastric phase.
- Intestinal phase.

Peptic ulcer

It is the term referred to the breakdown of the mucosal epithelium of stomach/duodenum.

Causes

- Disruption of mucosal barrier of GIT by infection, alcohol, drugs.
- Hypersecretion of acid (excess of smoking, alcohol).

Functions of gastric juice

1. The gastric juice contains proteolytic enzyme which helps in the digestion of proteins.
2. The intrinsic factor plays an important role in erythropoiesis.
3. The mucus present in the gastric juice protects the stomach wall from mechanical and chemical injury as well as from the digestive action of pepsin and hydrochloric acid.
4. Hydrochloric acid kills the bacteria entering the stomach.

Pancreatic Secretion

Composition

- Daily secretion: 1200–1500 ml/day.
- pH: 7.8–8.4 (alkaline pH helps to neutralize gastric acidity).

Electrolytes

Na^+, K^+, HCO_3^-, Cl^-

Enzymes

- Pancreatic α-amylase.
- Pancreatic lipase.
- Pancreatic esterase.
- Pancreatic phospholipase.
- Proteolytic enzymes.
- Trypsinogen, chymotrypsinogen, caboxypeptidase, ribonuclease.

Functions of pancreatic juice

- Pancreatic juice has important digestive and neutralizing functions.
- It plays an important role in the digestion of carbohydrates, proteins and lipids.
- Pancreatic juice contains bicarbonate enzymes which neutralize the acidity of chyme entering the intestine.

Bile

Composition

- Volume: 500–1000 ml/day.
- pH : 7.8–8.6.
- Water 97%.
- Bile salts.
- Bilirubin.
- Cholesterol.
- Fatty acids.
- Lecithin.

Electrolytes

Na^+, K^+, Ca^{2+}, Cl^-, HCO_3^-

Functions of Bile

- Bile salts help in digestion and absorption of fats and fat soluble vitamins (A, D, E, K).
- Neutralization of acid entering intestine from the stomach.
- Excretion of drugs, toxins, bile pigments, hormones, inorganic substances, cholesterol and lecithin.
- Bile has a laxative action and stimulates peristalsis.

Liver Function Tests (LFTs)

LFTs helps to diagnose hepatic damage:
The following tests are done to investigate the functional capacity of liver.

1. ***Plasma protein concentration:***

Total plasma concentration	6.4–8.3 gm/dL
S. Albumin	3–5 gm/dL
S. Globulin	2–3 gm/dL

S. Fibrinogen 0.3 gm/dl
S. Prothrombin 40 mg/dl
(A/G ratio) albumin/globulin ratio = 1.7 : 1.0

2. ***Liver enzyme estimation***
   - S. Alkaline phosphate (normal 5–13 kÅ)
   - SGOT, SGPT (normal 5–40 units)
3. ***Blood urea*** (20–40 mg/dl)
4. ***For lipid metabolism***

   Lipid profile

S. Cholesterol	Normal	120–200 mg/dL
S. Triglycerides	Normal	30–150 mg/dL

5. ***For carbohydrate metabolism***
   - Galactose tolerance test
   - Blood glucose; normal fasting blood glucose is 70–90 mg/dl.
6. ***For protein metabolism***
   Blood amino acid level: Normal 30–60 m/dL.
7. ***For assessing bile secretory function***
   - Total serum bilirubin: Normal: 0.2–0.8 mg/dL
   - Assessing detoxification function of liver
   - Hippuric acid excretion test
   - Bromosulphalein (BSP) excretion test
8. ***Ultrasound:*** It is useful technique for diagnosis liver cysts, abscess, and dilated hepatic ducts.
9. ***CT scan:*** Same as can be diagnosed by ultrasound.
10. ***Liver biopsy:*** For histocytological studies.

Review Questions

1. Give in short the functions of various parts of GIT.
2. Write short notes on:
   a. Salivary secretion and its function.
   b. Composition of pancreatic secretion and its function.
   c. Functions and composition of bile.
   d. Liver function tests.
   e. Functions of small intestine.
   f. Functions of large intestine.
   g. Defecation reflex.

7 Excretory System

KIDNEY

The **kidneys** are bean-shaped organs that lie in the abdominal cavity attached to the dorsal wall on either side of the spine at the level of T12 to L1 vertebrae. An artery from the dorsal aorta called the **renal artery** supplies blood to them and the **renal vein** drains them. A cavity within the kidney called the **pelvis** collects the urine and carries it to the **ureter**, which connects with the **bladder** where the urine is stored temporarily. Rings of muscle **(sphincters)** control the release of urine from the bladder and the urine leaves the body through the **urethra** (Fig. 7.1).

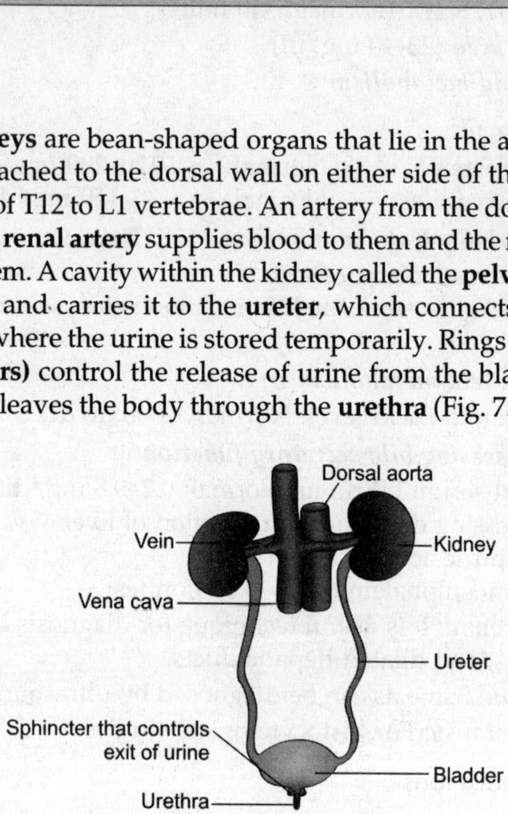

Fig. 7.1: Kidney

Functions of Kidney

- Excretion of metabolic waste products
- Maintains the normal hydrogen ion concentration of body fluids.
- Maintains water balance of the body and thereby plasma volume.

- Elimination of drugs and various other toxic substances from the body.
- Regulation of blood pressure in emergency conditions through liberation of renin from the juxtaglomerular apparatus.
- Regulation of erythropoiesis by formation of erythropoietin.
- Plays an important role in vitamin D metabolism.

Nephrons are the structural and functional units of the kidneys. Two kidneys have together about two million nephrons (Fig. 7.2).

Nephron consists of two major parts:
1. The glomerulus.
2. Renal tubule.

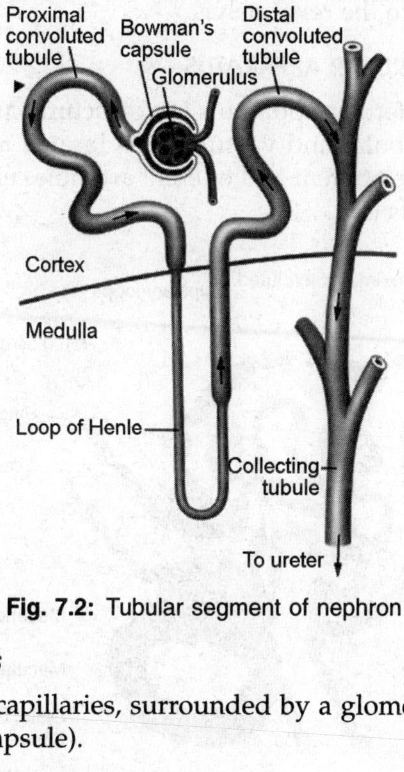

Fig. 7.2: Tubular segment of nephron

1. Glomerulus

It is a tuft of capillaries, surrounded by a glomerular capsule (Bowman's capsule).

Structure of glomerular membrane

It consists of the following layers:

- The endothelial cell layer of the capillaries.
- The basement membrane.
- The epithelial cells of the Bowman's capsule.

2. Renal Tubule

It is mainly formed of the following parts:

- Proximal convoluted tubule (PCT).
- Loop of Henle consisting of descending limb and ascending limb.
- Distal convoluted tubules. Its cells get modified to form the juxtaglomerular apparatus. The distal convoluted tubules join to form the collecting duct.
- The collecting ducts collect filtrate from many nephrons, and empty it into the renal pelvis.

JUXTAGLOMERULAR APPARATUS

The juxtaglomerular apparatus is a structural arrangement of specialized tubular and vascular cells located at the vascular pole where the afferent and efferent arterioles enter and leave the glomerulus (Fig. 7.3).

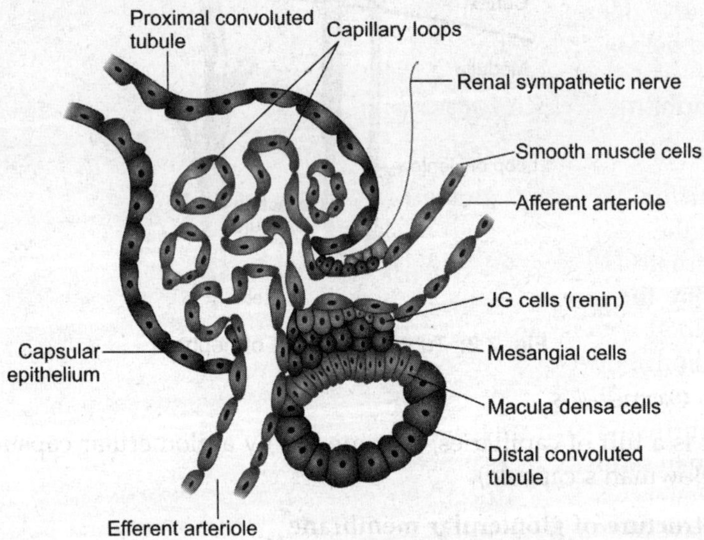

Fig. 7.3: Juxtaglomerular apparatus

There are 3 different types of cells in the juxtaglomerular apparatus: Granular juxtaglomerular cells, macula densa cells and mesangial cells.

1. ***Juxtaglomerular cells (JG cells):*** They are modified vascular smooth muscle cells. These cells function as baroreceptors.

   The juxtaglomerular cells synthesize, store and secrete renin.

   Renin is a glycoprotein. It acts on angiotensinogen of blood and converts it into angiotensin I. Angiotensin I is converted into angiotensin II by converting enzyme in the lungs.

   Angiotensin has the following functions:
   - It causes constriction of systemic arterioles causing elevation of blood pressure.
   - It stimulates adrenal cortex to secrete aldosterone.
   - It helps to maintain GFR.
2. ***Macula densa cells***
   - Macula densa cells are columnar epithelium thickening of the distal tubule.
   - They function as chemo receptors.
3. ***Mesangial cells:*** Mesangial cells are structural cells in the glomerulus that under normal conditions serve as anchors for the glomerular capillaries. They are contractile in nature and helps in regulating glomerular filtration.

Mechanisms of Urine Formation (Fig. 7.4)

Step 1: **Glomerular filtration**

Definition: Volume of glomerular filtrate formed each minute by all the nephrons in both the kidneys.

Normal: 125 ml/min = 180 litres/day.

Urine formation begins with the process of **filtration.** As the blood courses through the glomeruli, much of its fluid, containing both useful chemicals and dissolved waste materials, soaks out of the blood through the membranes (by osmosis and diffusion) where it is filtered and then flows into the Bowman's capsule. This process is called **glomerular filtration**. The water, waste products, salt, glucose, and other chemicals that have been filtered out of the blood are known collectively as glomerular filtrate. The glomerular filtrate consists primarily

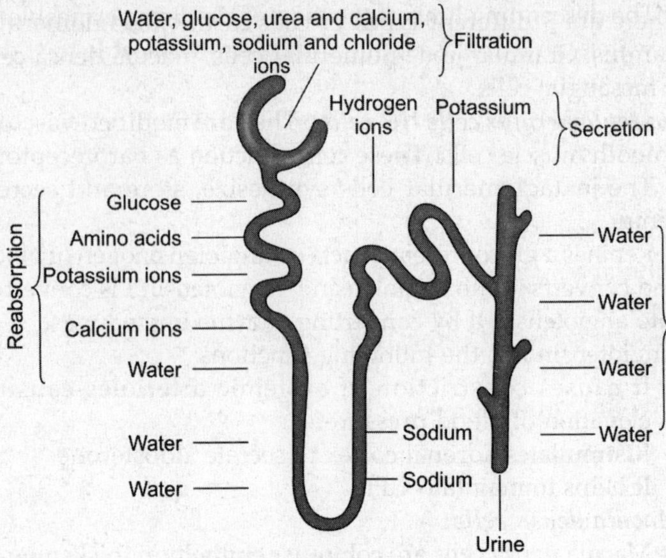

Fig. 7.4: Urine formation

of water, excess salts (primarily Na^+ and K^+), glucose, and a waste product of the body called **urea.**

Glomerular filtration rate is held relatively constant through intrinsic autoregulatory mechanisms, and extrinsic hormonal and neural mechanisms.

Step 2: **Tubular reabsorption**

1. Tubular reabsorption begins as soon as the filtrate enters the proximal convoluted tubule, and involves near total reabsorption of organic nutrients, reabsorption of water and ions.
2. The most abundant cation of the filtrate is Na^+.
3. Secondary active transport is responsible for absorption of glucose, amino acids, vitamins, and most cations, and occurs when solutes are cotransported with Na^+ when it moves along its concentration gradient.
4. Substances that are not reabsorbed or incompletely reabsorbed remain in the filtrate (urea, creatinine, and uric acid):
   a. The proximal convoluted tubule is most active in reabsorption.

b. The descending limb of the loop of Henle is permeable to water, while the ascending limb is impermeable to water but permeable to electrolytes.
c. The distal convoluted tubule and collecting ducts are permeable to Na^+ and water. Water permeability is regulated by the, antidiuretic hormone (Table 7.1).

Step 3: **Tubular secretion**

1. Tubular secretion disposes of unwanted solutes, rids the body of excess K^+, and controls blood pH.
2. Tubular secretion is most active in the proximal convoluted tubule, but occurs in the collecting ducts and distal convoluted tubules, as well.

Step 4: **Formation of concentrated urine** occurs in response to the release of antidiuretic hormone, which makes the collecting ducts permeable to water and increases water uptake from the urine.

In summary, three processes occurring in successive portions of the nephron accomplish the function of urine formation:

1. Filtration of water and dissolved substances out of the blood in the glomeruli and into Bowman's capsule.
2. Reabsorption of water and dissolved substances out of the kidney tubules back into the blood.
3. Secretion of hydrogen ions (H^+), potassium ions (K^+), ammonia (NH_3), and certain drugs out of the blood and into the kidney tubules, where they are eventually eliminated in the urine. Kidney tubule secretion plays a crucial role in maintaining the body's acid–base balance.

Micturition

Definition

Micturition is the process of accumulation of formed urine in the urinary bladder and evacuation of the same from the bladder from time to time, which are controlled by nervous mechanisms.

Urinary bladder stores the urine which is transported to it from the kidneys via the ureters. When the bladder is filled by the urine coming from the ureters, the intravesical pressure (pressure inside the bladder) increases. The bladder wall is

Table 7.1: Reabsorption capabilities of different segments of the renal tubules and collection ducts

Tubule segment	*Substance reabsorbed*	*Machanism*
Proximal convoluted tubule		
	Sodium ions (Na^+)	Primary active transport via basolateral Na^+ K^+ pump; sets up electrochemical gradient for passive solute diffusion, osmosis, and secondary active transport (cotransport) with Na^+
	Virtually all nutrients (glucose, amino acids, vitamins)	Secondary active transport with Na^+
	Cations (K^+, Mg^{2+}, and others)	Passive transport driven by electrochemical gradient for most; the paracellular route is important
	Anions (Cl^-, HCO_3^-)	Passive transport; paracellular diffusion driven by electrochemical gradient for Cl^- ; secondary active transport (with Na^+) for HCO_3^-
	Water	Osmosis; driven by solute reabsorption (obligatory)
	Uria and lipid-soluble solutes	Passive diffusion driven by the concentration gradient created by reabsorption of water
	Small proteins	Endocytosed by tubule cells and digested to amino acids within tubule cells
Loop of Henle		
Descending limb	Water	Osmosis
Ascending limb	Na^+, Cl^-, K^+	Secondary active transport of Cl^- , Na^+, and K^+ via Na^+ -K^+-$2Cl^-$ cotransporter in thick portion; paracellular diffusion; Na^+ -H^+ antiport
	Ca^{2+}, Mg^{2+}	Passive paracellular diffusion driven by electrochemical gradient.

Contd.

Table 7.1: Reabsorption capabilities of different segments of the renal tubules and collection ducts (*contd.*)

Tubule segment	*Substance reabsorbed*	*Machanism*
Distal convoluted tuble		
	Na^+, Cl^-	Primary active Na^+ transport at basolateral membrane; secondary active transport at luminal membrane via Na^+-Cl^- symporter and channels; aldosterone-regulated at distal portion
	Ca^{2+}	Passive uptake via PTH-modulated channels in luminal membrane; primary and secondary active transport (antiport with Na^+) in basolateral membrane
Collecting duct		
	Na^+, H^+ K^+, HCO_3^-, Cl^-	Primary active transport of Na^+ (requires aldosterone) and the medullary gradient create the conditions for passive transport of some HCO_3^- and Cl^- and cotransport of H^+, Cl^-, and HCO_3^-; K^+ is both reabsorbed and secreted (aldosterone dependent), usually resulting in net K^+ secretion
	Water	Osmosis; controlled (facultative) water reabsorption; ADH required to insert aquaporins
	Urea	Facilitated diffusion in response to concentration gradient in the deep medulla region; recycles and contributes to medullary osmotic gradient

stretched, and the stretch receptors in the wall are stimulated. Sensory signals are conducted to the sacral segments of the spinal cord through the pelvic nerves and then through the parasympathetic fibres in the same nerve to the bladder wall which causes contraction of the detrusor muscle of bladder and relaxation of the internal sphincter and emptying of the bladder. This is the micturition reflex. First urge to pass urine is felt at 150 ml urine volume. Initiation of micturition reflex is at 400 ml urine volume.

Renal Function Tests

1. **Urine examination:**

Colour: pale yellow.

Composition

Inorganic : Na^+,K^+,Ca^{2+}, phosphate.
Organic : Urea, uric acid, creatinine.
Volume : 1–2.5 litres/day (average 1.5 litres/day).
Oliguria : Urine volume <400 ml/day.
Anuria : Urine volume <100 ml/day.
Polyuria : Urine volume >2.5 litres/day.
Specific gravity : 1001–1040.
Reaction : 4.5–8.0 (6–6.5, slight acidic).

Microscopic examination

- 1–2 WBC or pus cells/HPF: normal.
- Presence of granular casts, RBCs, bacteria, glucose, albumin and ketone bodies are abnormal (Table 7.2).

2. **Analysis of blood**
   - Blood urea (norma 20–40 mg).
   - Plasma ceatinine (normal 0.6–1.5 mg%).
   - Serum proteins (norma 6.7–8 mg%).
   - Serum cholesterol (150–200 mg%).
3. **Clearance test to measure GFR:** Glomerular filtration rate can be accurately measured by renal clearance test.
   - Inulin clearance test.
   - Creatinine clearance test.
   - Urea clearance test.

Table 7.2: Abnormal urinary constituents

Substance	*Name of condition*	*Possible causes*
Glucose	Glycosuria	Nonpathological; excessive intake of sugary foods
Proteins	Proteinuria, or albuminuria	Nonpathological; excessive physical exertion; pregnancy; high-protein diet Pathological (over 250 mg/day): heart failure, severe hypertension; glomerulonephritis; often initial sign of asymptomatic renal disease
Ketone bodies	Ketonuria	Excessive formation and accumulation of ketone bodies, as in starvation and untreated diabetes mellitus
Hemoglobin	Hemoglobinuria	Various: transfusion reaction, hemolytic anemia, severe burns, etc.
Bile pigments	Bilirubinuria	Liver disease (hepat itis, cirrhosis) or obstruction of bile ducts from liver or gallbladder
Erythrocytes	Hematuria	Bleeding urinary tract (due to trauma, kidney stones, infection, or neoplasm)
Leukocytes (pus)	Pyuria	Urinary tract infection

The inulin clearance, thus GFR is calculated by the formula:

C_{in} (GFR)= $U_{in} \times V/P_{in}$

Where

C_{in} inulin clearance

U_{in} urine concentration of inulin in mg/ml

V urine flow rate ml/min

P_{in} plasma concentration of inulin in mg/ml

4. **PSP (phenolsulfonephthalein) excretion test** is used to assess tubular function.
5. **Radiology**
   - Plain radiograph of abdomen is useful in detecting renal stones.
   - Intravenous pyelography (IVP) is useful to study the size, shape and position of the kidney.

- *Ultrasonography:* Non invasive, methods to evaluate size, shape, position of kidney and to detect tumor, stones, etc. of the kidney, ureter, bladder.
- Computed tomography (CT) is performed to detect abnormalities as mentioned in USG.

Review Questions

1. Enumerate the functions of kidney.
2. Describe the mechanism of urine formation.
3. Write in brief the different renal function tests.
4. Write short notes on:
   - Micturition.
   - Juxtaglomerular apparatus.
   - Glomerular filtration.
   - Nephron.

8 Endocrine System

Endocrines are also called ductless glands which secrete physiologically active substances called hormones directly into the blood.

Hormones

Definition: Secretary products of endocrine glands released directly into the circulation in small amounts in response to a specific stimulus and produce response on the target cells.

There are three major classes of hormones

1. *Steroids:* Adrenal cortical hormones, males and female steroids hormones.
2. *Proteins or polypeptides:* Hormones of pituitary, hypothalamus and pancreas.
3. *Amino acid derivatives:* Thyroid hormones, adrenal medullary hormones.

Major Endocrine Glands

Hypothalamus

Hypothalamus secretes various releasing and inhibitory hormones:

- Growth hormone releasing hormone (GHRH).
- Corticotropin releasing hormone (CRH).
- Thyroid releasing hormone (TRH).
- Gonadotropin releasing hormone (GnRH).
- Growth hormone inhibitory hormone (GHIH).

Pituitary Glands

- Thyroid stimulating hormone (TSH).
- Adrenocorticotropic hormone (ACTH).
- Growth hormone (GH).

- Follicle stimulating hormone (FSH).
- Luteinizing hormone (LH).
- Antidiuretic hormone (ADH).
- Oxytocin.

Thyroid

- Thyroxine (T4).
- Triiodothyronine (T3).
- Calcitonin.

Parathyroid

Parathyroid hormone

Adrenal Gland

- *Cortex:* Mineralocorticoids (aldosterone), glucocorticoids (cortisol).
- *Medulla:* Epinephrine, norepinephrine.

Pancreas

Insulin, glucagon.

Ovaries

Oestrogen, progesterone

Testis

Testosterone

Mechanism of Hormonal Action

There are basic three mechanisms of hormone action:

1. Activation of intracellular enzyme.
2. Activation of genes.
3. Change in the membrane permeability.

Hormones of pituitary gland:

Growth Hormone

GH is a single polypeptide containing 191 amino acids.

Actions

GH causes the growth of almost all the tissues of the body.

1. On Protein Metabolism

Anabolic–stimulates protein synthesis it increases transport of amino acids.

2. Fat Metabolism

- Increases mobilization of fat from adipose tissue.
- Increases the level of circulating free fatty acids.
- Increases hepatic oxidation of fatty acids to ketone bodies.

3. On Carbohydrate Metabolism

Diabetogenic effect:

- Enhances glycogen deposition in the cell.
- Decrease utilization, of glucose by the cell and increases blood glucose level.

4. Stimulation of Growth of Bone, Cartilage and Connective Tissue

Effect of growth hormone on bones and cartilages are mediated by growth factors called somatomedins which are synthesized by liver. Before epiphysial closure long bones increase in length. After epiphysial closure the bones thickness increases.

Stimulation of GH secretion

- GHRH.
- Stress, trauma.
- Exercise, fasting, hypoglycemia.

Inhibition

- GHIH.
- Glucose.
- Glucocorticoids.
- Increases FFA.

Applied

Gigantism: It is the over secretion of GH before adolescence.

Features

- Excessive increase in the length of long bones.
- Person becomes a giant may grow to a height of 6–8 feet.
- Large hands and feet.
- Hyperglycemia.

Acromegaly

- Excessive GH secretion during adulthood (i.e. after fusion of epiphysis).
- Person cannot grow taller but bones continue to grow in thickness.
- Elongation and widening of mandible (prognathism).
- Acromegalic facies; thickness of skin and coarsening of facial features.
- Growth of vertebrae-kyphosis.
- Organomegaly (liver, kidney, greatly enlarged).

Dwarfism

This results from the decreased secretion of GH during childhood. There is stunted physical growth. The mental growth of pituitary dwarf is normal.

Oxytocin

It is a polypeptide hormone containing nine amino acids. It is synthesized by paraventricular nucleus of hypothalamus and stored in the post pituitary.

Action

- Oxytocin powerfully stimulates the pregnant uterus especially towards the end of gestation and plays a role in labour.
- Oxytocin facilitates the transport of sperm in the female genital tract.
- Oxytocin causes contraction of myoepithelial cells of lactating mammary glands which leads to expression of milk from alveoli into the ducts, so that the baby can obtain it by suckling. This is known as the milk down reflex.

Stimuli for release of oxytocin:

- Suckling by the baby.
- Distension of cervix and vagina.

ADH: It is a polypeptide hormone containing 9 amino acids.

It is synthesized in the supraoptic nucleus of hypothalamus and stored in the posterior pituitary.

Control of secretion

Increase secretion:

- Hyperosmolarity of ECF (extracellular fluid).
- Water deprivation.
- Pain, stress.
- Hypoxia.

Decrease secretion:

- Hyposmolality of ECF.
- Increase in blood pressure.

Role of ADH

- It stimulates reabsorption of water by the distal convoluted and the collecting renal tubules and thus regulates urine volume.
- In high dose it causes constriction of blood vessels and increases blood pressure.

Diabetes insipidus:

- It is a disease caused by decrease or lack of ADH.
- It is characterized by increased formation of urine of low specific gravity.

Features

- Polyuria.
- Polydipsia.

Thyroid Gland

Thyroid gland consists of about three million of follicles. Each follicle is lined by epithelial cells and is filled with colloid. Colloid is made up glycoprotein called thyroglobulin. Thyroid hormones remain bound to thyroglobulin until their secretion.

Thyroid hormones

- Thyroxine T4.
- Triiodothyronine T3.
- Calcitonin.

Synthesis of thyroid hormones:

- Iodine is required for synthesis of thyroid hormones
- The requirement of iodine is 1 mg/week.

Formation of thyroid hormone is by the following steps:

1. *Oxidation of iodine ion:* The basal membrane of thyroid gland has an iodide pump, which pumps iodide actively into the interior of the cell which is then oxidized to iodine by enzyme peroxidase.
2. *Iodination of tyrosine*
   Oxidized iodine binds with amino acid tyrosine.
   Tyrosine is first oxidized to MIT (monoiodotyrosine
   Tyrosine is then oxidized to DIT (diiodotyrosine)
   Then
   MIT + DIT = T_3 (triiodothyronine)
   DIT + DIT = T_4 (thyroxine)
3. Storage of hormones, after formation T3 and T4 are stored in the thyroglobulin molecule.

Actions of Thyroid Hormones

Growth and development

Thyroid hormone is necessary for normal body growth and skeletal maturation. It helps in myelination and plays an essential role in growth and development of central nervous system.

On metabolism

- T_3 and T_4 increase the metabolic activity of almost all the cells in the body and increase BMR.
- T_3 and T_4 increase the number and activity of mitochondria and ATP synthesis.

Carbohydrate metabolism

Thyroid hormones increase the absorption of glucose from intestine. It also stimulates the utilization of glucose.

Protein metabolism

In physiological doses thyroid hormone increases and protein synthesis. In high concentration there is catabolic effect leading to muscle weakness, fatiguability and decreases bone mass.

Fat metabolism

- Thyroid hormones lead to mobilization of fat from adipose tissue and increase levels of fatty acids in the blood.
- They also increase excretion of cholesterol in bile.

Effect on cardiovascular system

- Thyroid hormone increases HR, CO and arterial pressure.
- Moderate increase in thyroid hormones increase the strength of heart but in excessive doses due to excess protein catabolism there occurs decrease in heart muscular strength.

Effect on respiratory system

The rate and depth of respiration is increased under the influence of thyroid hormones.

GIT

Thyroid hormones increase the rate of secretion of digestive juices and motility of GIT.

Reproductive system

- It is important for normal gonadal development.
- In females lack of thyroid hormone increases menstrual bleeding whereas excess, leads to scanty menstruation.

TSH (Thyroid Stimulating Hormone)

It increases the releases of T3, T4 from the thyroid gland by the following:

- Increase release of thyroid hormones by the cells.
- Increase activity of iodide pump.
- Increase iodination of tyrosine.
- Increase size and secretary activity of thyroid cells.

Regulation of Thyroid Hormones

There is negative feedback mechanism which regulates thyroid hormones:

Goiter

Enlargement of thyroid gland is called **goiter**.

Increase thyroid hormones in the body fluids

↓

Decrease rate of secretion of TSH by anterior pituitary

↓

Decrease release and synthesis of thyroid hormones

Causes

- Iodide deficiency.
- Thyroiditis.
- Abnormalities in the enzymes system required for thyroid hormones synthesis.
- Presence of goitrogenic substances (cabbage, turnip, etc.) in the food.

It results in hypothyroidism where T3 and T4 levels are decreased in the blood.

Features of hypothyroidism **(myoxedema)**

Fatigue

- Sleeping for 14–16 hours.
- Muscular sluggishness.
- Cold intolerance.
- Low BMR.
- Decrease growth of hair, scaliness of skin.
- Frog like husky voice.
- Bagginess under the eyes and swelling of face.

Cretinism

Children or infants who are hypothyroid during fetal life, infancy and childhood.

Causes

Maternal iodine deficiency.

Features

- Stunted skeletal growth.
- Deformed bone and teeth.
- Rough dry skin, scanty hairs.
- Growth of sex organs retarded.
- Mental retardation.

Hyperthyroidism

- Common cause-autoimmune disorder—Grave's diseases (exophthalmic goitre) or thyrotoxicosis
- It is mostly due to development of thyroid stimulating antibodies in the blood.

Features

- Increase BMR.
- Heat intolerance.
- Weight loss.
- Diarrhoea, muscular weakness, fatigue.
- Inability to sleep.
- Increase HR, systolic BP.
- Eye signs—exophthalmos (protusion of eyeballs).
- Thyroid diabetes.

Parathyroid

- Parathyroid glands (four small glands) are located behind the thyroid gland.
- It secretes parathyroid hormone (parathormone, PTH)
- It is a protein hormone.

Effect of PTH

Parathyroid hormone increases the rate of bone resorption with consequent mobilization of calcium and phosphate.

- PTH increases calcium and phosphate absorption from gut.
- PTH increases renal tubular reabsorption of calcium.
- It increases renal excretion of phosphate.
- PTH secretion is regulated by concentration of calcium in the blood. Increase in Ca^{2+} concentration inhibits the secretion whereas decreases in concentration stimulate secretion.

Along with vitamin D and calcitonin, it regulates serum calcium and serum phosphate levels.

Tetany (Hypoparathyroidism)

It occurs due to accidental removal of parathyroid glands during thyroidectomy.

Features

There is decrease in serum Ca^{2+} levels and neuromuscular hyperexcitability.

Clinical signs

- Facial irritability.
- Carpopedal spasm (Trousseau's sign).

Hyperparathyroidism

Causes

- Hyperplasia of parathyroid glands.
- Chronic renal disease.

Features

- Increase serum Ca^{2+} resulting in weakness, loss of muscle tone.
- Anorexia, nausea, vomiting, constipation.
- Kidney stones.
- Bones demineralisation leading to spontaneous fractures.

Calcitonin

- Calcitonin is a protein hormone synthesized by parafollicular cells presents between the thyroid follicles.
- Its effect is opposite to PTH.
- It inhibits the reabsorbtion of calcium and phosphate from GIT and bones and increases their renal excretion.
- Increase in serum calcium levels stimulates secretion of calcitonin which returns the calcium level back towards normal.

Vitamin D

- The principal active form of vitamin D is 1, 25-dihydroxy cholecalciferol (calcitriol) which regulates Ca^{2+} levels.
- It increases the mobilization of Ca^{2+} and phosphate from bone.
- It increases absorption of Ca^{2+} from GIT.
- It promotes Ca^{2+} reabsorption from kidney.

Rickets

It is a disease occurring in children as result of calcium and phosphate deficiency due to lack of vitamin D.

Features

- Deformed bones.
- Retarded growth.
- Short stature.
- Delayed dentition.

Osteomalacia

- It is rickets in adults due to deficiency of vitamin D and Ca^{2+} in diet.
- It results in decrease in mineralization of the bones. Fractures and myopathy is common.

Pancreas

Hormones of pancreas are:
- Insulin.
- Glucagon.

Glucagon

It is secreted by α cells of pancreas

Action

- Glucagon stimulates glycogenolysis, gluconeogenesis
- Increases fatty acids.

Glucagon secretion is increased by:
- Hypoglycemia.
- Stress.
- Protein meal.
- GIT hormones like gastrin.
- Muscular exercise.

Insulin

It is secreted by β cells of pancreas

Action

- Insulin increases uptake of glucose into muscles and most of the other tissues in the body except kidney, RBC.
- Insulin produces hypoglycemia by:
  - Increasing utilization of glucose.
  - Increase glycogen synthesis.

- Insulin increases synthesis of free fatty acids and triglycerides in muscles, adipose tissue and liver.
- It also increase protein synthesis.
- It is the hormone of energy storage.

Regulation of insulin secretion

Increase in release is by

- Blood sugar, amino acids.
- GIT hormones like gastrin.

Decrease in release is by

- Starvation.
- Sympathetic stimulation.

Diabetes Mellitus

Diabetes mellitus is a decrease resulting from decreased secretion of insulin.

It is of two types:

1. Insulin dependent diabetes mellitus/Type I.
2. Noninsulin dependent diabetes mellitus/Type II.

Features

- Increases in blood glucose.
- Loss of glucose in urine.
- Depletion of proteins.
- Polyuria.
- Polydipsia.
- Polyphagia.
- Weight loss.

Adrenal Cortex

- There are two adrenal glands lying at the superior poles of the kidneys. It has two parts.
- Outer-adrenal cortex.
- Inner–adrenal medulla.

Adrenal cortex has three zones which produce following hormones:

- Zona glomerulosa–mineralocorticoids.
- Zona fasiculata–glucocorticoids.
- Zona reticularis–sex steroids.

Adrenal Medulla Secretes

Adrenaline and noradrenaline.

Mineralocortcoids

Most potent mineralocorticoid is **aldosterone**.

Functions of aldosterone

- Aldosterone causes increased absorption of sodium and excretion of potassium from renal tubules.
- It helps in regulation of extracellular fluid volume.
- It also increases sodium absorption from GIT, sweat and salivary glands.

Applied

- **Addison's disease** (primary adrenocortical insufficiency).
- Addison's disease is due to decreased secretion of adrenocortical hormones.

Features

- Decreased blood pressure.
- Anorexia, nausea, vomiting, diarrhea, dehydration, weight loss.
- Muscular weakness.
- Generalized pigmentation of skin.
- Decreased ability to withstand stress.

Glucocorticoids

Most potent glucocorticoid is **cortisol**

Functions of cortisol

- Cortisol stimulates gluconeogenesis and increases blood glucose level.
- Corisol decreases protein synthesis and increase catabolism of proteins.
- It increases free fatty acid levels in the body.
- Cortisol also has important anti-inflammatory and anti-allergic effect.
- It increases the resistance to stress.

Cushing Syndrome

Hypersecretion of cortisol causes cushing syndrome

Features

- Moonface.
- Buffalo lump.
- Hypertension.
- Increase blood glucose level.
- Muscular weakness.
- Osteoporosis.
- Weakness in bones.
- Suppressed immune system.

Review Questions

1. Mention the different endocrine glands and the hormones.
2. Enumerate the functions of growth hormone
3. Write in brief the functions of thyroid hormone
4. Give the functions of insulin
5. Write the functions of cortisol
6. Write short notes on:
   a. Acromegaly
   b. Dwarfism
   c. Cushing syndrome
   d. Addison's disease
   e. Goitre

9 Reproduction

MALE REPRODUCTIVE SYSTEM

The male reproductive system constituted by the following:

Testis

Functions

- Production and storage of sperms.
- Synthesis and secretion of testosterone.

Epididymis

Functions

- Storage of sperms.
- Its secretion nourishes the sperms and helps them to mature.
- Sperms acquires motility in the epididymis.

Vas Deferens

Serves as a secondary store house for sperms which are released at the time of ejaculation.

Seminal Vesicles

Its secretion contributes 60% of total volume of semen and also provides energy for the movement of sperm.

Prostate

It secretes prostatic fluid which contributes to 20% of total volume of semen.

Bulbourethral Glands

Functions

- Lubrication.
- Alkalinity helps to protect the sperms.

Testosterone

- Synthesized from cholesterol in the testis.
- Small amount by adrenal cortex.

Action

1. Helps in spermatogenesis.
2. Responsible for development of epididymis, seminal vesicles, prostate, penis and secondary sexual characters at puberty in males.
3. It increases the synthesis of proteins and muscular strength.
4. Increases the thickness of bones and helps in deposition of Ca^{2+} salts.
5. Increases BMR.
6. Increases erythropoiesis.

Spermatogenesis

- The process of formation of sperms is known as spermatogenesis.
- It occurs in the testis.
- Duration – 74 days.

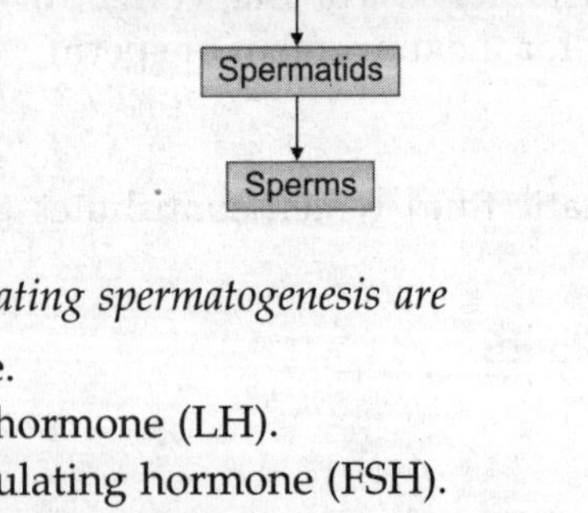

Hormones regulating spermatogenesis are

1. Testosterone.
2. Luteinizing hormone (LH).
3. Follicle stimulating hormone (FSH).
4. Growth hormone.

Semen

- It is also called seminal fluid.
- It contains—sperms and secretion of seminal tract, prostate gland.
- Color—White.
- Volume—2.5–3.5 ml/ejaculate.
- Sperm count—80–120 millions/ml.
- Reaction–alkaline
- Rich in fructose which provides nourishment to the sperms.

FEMALE REPRODUCTIVE SYSTEM

Female reproductive system includes:

1. Uterus
2. Vagina
3. Fallopian tubes
4. Ovary.

Uterus

Function

The uterine endometrium undergoes characteristic changes during menstrual cycle. Uterus plays an important role in maintaining growth and development of embryo.

Fallopian Tube

Functions

- Provides passage by which ova can reach the uterus.
- Site of fertilization.

Ovary

Functions

- Production of ovum.
- Secretion of female hormones (oestrogen and progesterone).

Female Hormones

Oestrogen

Sources

- The ovaries.
- Placenta.

- Adrenal cortex (small amount).

Action

- Promotes the growth and development of ovaries, uterus, vagina and fallopian tubes.
- It promotes the motility of fallopian tube which plays an important role in transport of sperms.
- Oestrogen is responsible for the development of female secondary sexual characters.
- It is responsible for the proliferative stage of menstruation.
- Oestrogen causes increase in osteoblastic activity and increase in growth spurt at puberty.
- It causes protein deposition.
- Oestrogen causes increased fat deposition in subcutaneous tissue and also in other particular regions to make a typical feminine body.
- It causes growth of uterus during pregnancy.

Progesterone

Sources

- Ovaries.
- Placenta.
- Adrenal cortex (small amount).

Action

- Progesterone is responsible for premenstrual changes of uterine mucosa.
- It prepares the endometrium of uterus for implantation of fertilized ovum.
- Progesterone causes development of lobules and alveoli of the breast.
- It increases the basal body temperature slightly.

Menstrual Cycle

- Cyclic discharge of blood, mucous and certain other substances from the uterus in the reproductive life of the females, at an average interval of 28 days (24–32) is called menstruation.

- It is absent before puberty, during pregnancy and after menopause.

Composition

- Blood (30—40 ml).
- Stripped of endometrium.
- Mucus.
- Leukocytes.

Phases

1. Menstrual phase.
2. Proliferative phase.
3. Secretory phase.

Menstrual Phase

- If the ovum is not fertilized, bleeding from the female genital tract occurs which lasts for about 3–5 days.
- Most of the endometrium is sheded, only basal layer remains intact. Capillaries rupture and haemorrhage occurs.
- Lack of progesterone is the main cause.

Duration

3–5 days

Proliferative Phase

- During proliferative phase oestrogens are secreted in large quantities.
- There is regeneration of the endometrium. There is growth of the blood vessels and glands. Mucosa thickens and becomes more vascular.

Duration

5—14 days

Secretory Phase

During this phase both oestrogen and progesterone are secreted in large quantities, progesterone prepares the endometrium for implantation of the fertilized ovum. There is increase in gland size and blood supply.

Duration

14 days

If no fertilization takes places, there is sharp decrease in progesterone and oestrogen and new cycle begins.

Review Questions

Write short notes on:

a. Testosterone
b. Oestrogens and progesterones
c. Menstrual cycle
d. Spermatogenesis.

10 Special Senses

THE EYE (VISION) (Fig. 10.1)

Physiological Anatomy

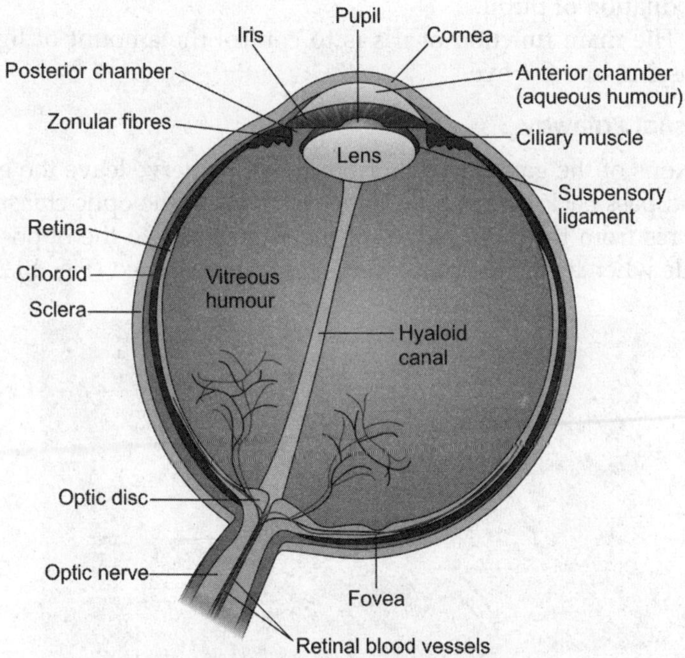

Fig. 10.1: Structure of eye

Eyeball is spherical, 24 mm in diameter having three layers:

1. The outer layer made up of sclera and cornea.
2. Middle highly vascular layer made up of choroid, ciliary body and iris.
3. Inner nervous layer called **retina**.

Retina contains the photo receptors (rods and cones)

Optic disc is a small area of retina where optic nerve leaves the eye, it contains no photoreceptors. It is, therefore, called as blind spot where there is no perception of light.

Macula leuta marks the location of fovea centralis. It is the point of greatest visual acuity in the retina.

Muscles of the Iris

1. Sphincter pupillae muscle: Its contraction leads to constriction of pupil.
2. Dilator pupillae muscle: When this muscle contracts it causes dilation of pupil.

The main function of iris is to control the amount of light passing into the eye.

Visual Pathway

Axons of the ganglion cells from the optic nerve leave the eye and pass backwards at the optic chiasma. At the optic chiasma fibres from the nasal halves of the retina cross to the opposite side whereas the temporal fibres remain uncrossed (Fig. 10.2).

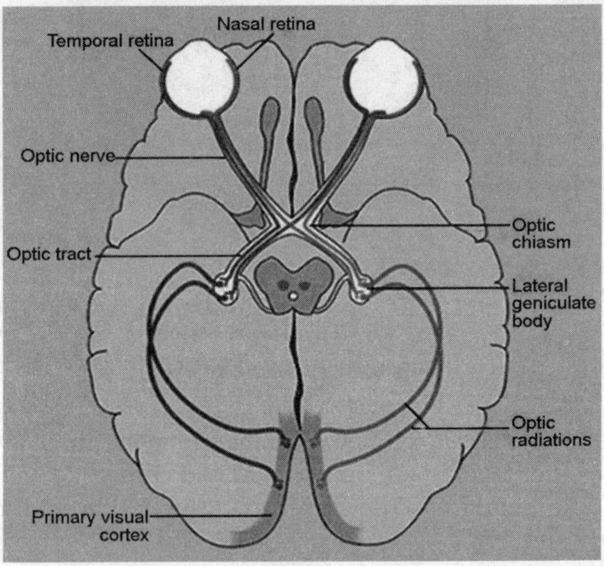

Fig. 10.2: Visual pathway

These fibers form the optic tract which ends in the lateral geniculate body (LGB).

From LGB the fibres pass by the way of optic radiations to primary visual cortex in the occipital lobe.

Primary visual area (area 17) it is the highest area for perception of visual sense.

Visual association area (areas 18, 19) is associated with interpretation, visual orientation and visual memory.

Image Forming Mechanism

1. The light rays from a distant object (more than 6 meters) that strike a lens are approximately parallel. The light rays from an object closer than 6 metres are diverging and therefore are brought to focus farther back on the principal axis than the principal focus.
2. Power of lens = 1/focal length of the lens (meters)
   Normal: 59 dioptres
3. The centre point of lens is called optical centre or nodal point.
4. The angle subtended by any object at the nodal point is called the visual angle.
5. Visual Acuity: It is the power of the eye to resolve two stimuli separately in space. It is the sharpness to which the details and contours of objects are perceived.
   For distant vision it is tested by Snellen's chart
   Near vision-jagcr's chart.

Factors Affecting Visual Acuity

1. It is low in defects of image forming mechanisms.
2. It is maximal at fovea centralis.
3. It is directly proportional to visual angle.
4. Stimulus factors like illumination, brightness also affect visual activity.

Defects of image forming mechanisms: **(Refractive errors of the eye).**

The normal eye with correct refraction is called emmetropic eye, any deviation from emmetropia is called ametropia. They are briefly given below (Fig. 10.3).

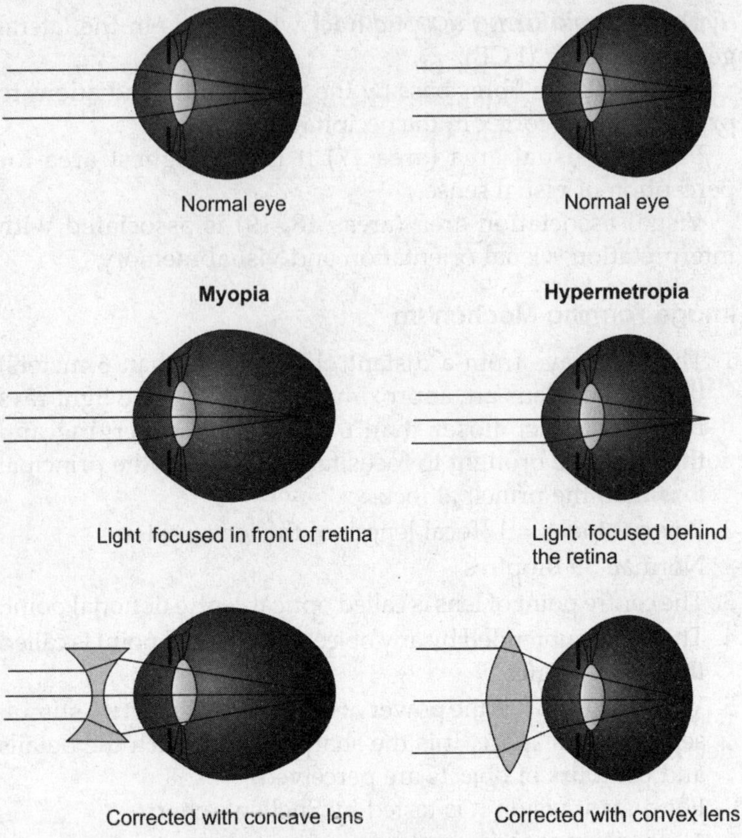

Fig. 10.3: Refractive errors

Myopia *(Short sightedness)*

Myopia is the refractive error of the eye in which the parallel rays coming from the distant object are focused in front of the retina.

The subject is able to see near object but the distant vision is diminished.

It is either due to:

- Too long eyeball
- Increased refractive power of the lens.

Correction: Concave lens.

Hypermetropia (Long sightedness)

It is the refractive error of the eye in which the parallel rays coming from the distant object are focused behind the retina. Person can see distant objects but not near ones.

It is either due to:
- Too Short eyeball
- Decreased refractive power of the lens.

Correction

Convex lens

Astigmatism

It is the refractive error of the eye in which the light rays are not brought to a point focus on the retina.

It is due to difference in horizontal and vertical curvature of cornea (irregular shape of cornea)

Correction

Cylindrical lens.

Presbyopia

It is the condition in which the ability of the eye to accommodate decreases with advancing age.

The lens of the eye loses its elasticity because of progressive denaturation of lens proteins.

Correction

Presbyopic person is given bifocal glasses with upper segment focused for seeing distant objects and lower segment focused for seeing near objects.

Accommodation

Definition

The ability of the eye to focus on object at varying distances is called accommodation.

Accommodation reflex (near response) consists of:
1. Contraction of ciliary muscles.
2. Constriction of pupil.
3. Convergence of visual axes.

Photochemistry of vision: Photoreceptors of eye are rods and cones.

Rods: They are responsible for vision in dim light (scotopic vision)

Cones: They are responsible for vision in bright light (photopic vision), colour sensation and acuity of vision.

Visibility Range

The eye responds to light of wavelengths between 400 nm to 750 nm. Beyond this range the photoreceptors are not stimulated. For this reason ultraviolet rays (below 400 nm) and infra red (above 750 nm) are not visible.

Colour Vision

The human eye can recognize about 150 different colours of the visible spectrum. It is mainly the function of cones.

Primary Colour

The primary colors are those which when combined together produce white. They are red, green and blue. When mixed in equal proportion they give white.

Complementary Colour

These are the pairs of two colors which produce white when mixed in proper proportion, e.g. red and greenish blue.

Young-Helmholtz Trichromatic Theory for Colour Vision

According to this theory, retina has three types of cones with three fundamental sensations- red, green and blue. These three types of cones contain three photochemical substance corresponding the three fundamental colour sensations. Each cone gives response to one of the primary colours-red, green and blue. The different colour sensations are produced by the stimulation of various combinations of the three types of cones. For the sensation of white all the three types of cones are stimulated equally.

Colour Blindness

- Colour blindness means defect or lack of appreciation of one or more colours.
- It is common in 8% of males and only 0.4% females.
- It is inherited as sex linked recessive disorder.

Colour Blindness Classification

It is based upon the Young-Helmholtz theory of colour vision.

Trichromats	**Dichromats**	**Monochromats**
Protanomaly	1. Protanopia	
Deuteranomly	2. Deuteranopia	
Tritanomaly	3. Tritanopia	

Anopia is colour blindness

Anomaly is color weakness.

1. ***Trichromats:*** These individuals can see all three colours but appreciation of one particular colour is weak. It is classified in to three categories.
   - *Protanomaly:* Red colour vision is subnormal.
   - *Deuteranomaly:* Green colour vision is subnormal.
   - *Tritanomaly:* Blue colour vision is subnormal.
2. ***Dichromats*:** Dichromats can appreciate only two colours but fail to see one.

   It is classified in to three groups:
   - *Protanopia:* Red colour cannot be appreciated
   - *Deuteranopia:* Green colour cannot be appreciated
   - *Tritanopia:* Blue colour cannot be appreciated.
3. ***Monochromats:*** They see only black and white shades of gray.

   Tests for detecting color vision:
   - Holmgren's wool test.
   - Ishihara's test
   - Edridge green lantern test.

Photochemical Changes in Rhodopsin

Visual Cycle

Visual purple or rhodopsin is the photosensitive pigment of the rod. It is bleached on exposure to light.

When light falls on retina, rhodopsin passes through several stages. It is first converted to lumirhodopsin and then to metarhodopsin. The metarhodopsin is then converted into retinine and protein called opsin. Retinine is the oxidative product of vitamin A and opsin is the protein of rhodopsin. The photo pigment must be regenerated after being bleached by light so as to prepare for another response. It can be synthesized directly from vitamin A (Fig. 10.4).

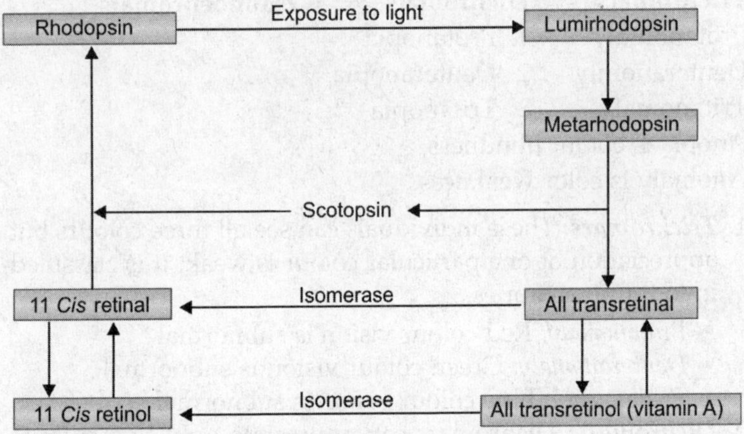

Fig. 10.4: Visual cycle

Dark Adaptation

Dark adaptation is the process by which the person is able to see the objects in dim light.

The dark adaptation is due to the following:

- Resynthesis of rhodopsin
- Dilation of pupil

Light Adaptation

Light adaptation is the process in which eyes gets adapted to light. When a person enters bright area from a dim light area he feels discomfort after some time the eye becomes adapted to light, he can see the objects without any discomfort.

Light adaptation is nothing but the disappearance of dark adaptation

Light adaptation is due to the following

- Breakdown of rhodopsin
- Constriction of pupil.

Night Blindness

Night Blindness is defined as the loss of vision in dim light.

Causes

It is due to deficiency of vitamin A, which is essential for function of rods.

Either due to

- Dietary deficiency
- Decrease absorption of vitamin A from intestine.

Retinal function can be restored if treatment is given with vitamin A.

Review Questions

1. Define visual acuity. Mention the refractive errors of eye.
2. Describe in brief about colour vision. Name the different tests done for colour vision.
3. Describe the photo chemistry of vision. Add a note on night blindness.
4. Write short notes on:
   a. Colour blindness.
   b. Dark adaptation.
   c. Visual cycle.

EAR

The ear consists of three parts external ear, middle ear and internal ear (Fig.10.5).

External Ear

It is formed by two parts:

- Auricle or pinna
- External auditory canal/meatus.

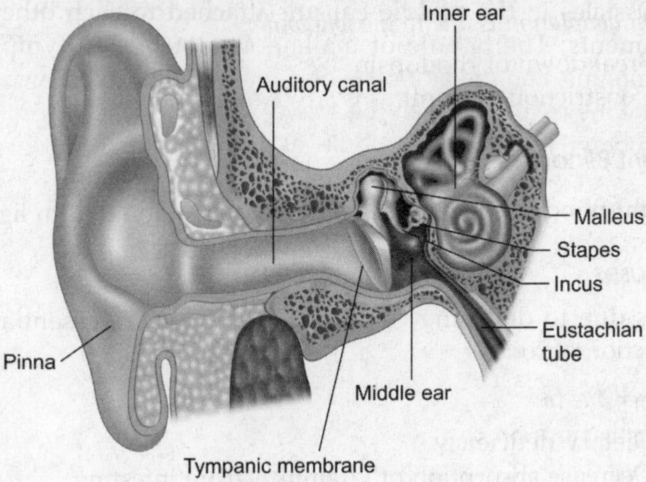

Fig. 10.5: Structure of ear

1. ***Auricle/Pinna:*** Pinna collects and reflects the sound waves into external auditory canal.
2. ***External auditory canal/meatus***
   - External auditory canal conducts the sound waves to the tympanic membrane
   - The hairs in the external auditory canal prevent the entry of foreign particles.

Middle Ear

It is an air filled cavity and separated from the external auditory canal by tympanic membrane.

It consists of the following structures:
- Auditory/ear ossicles
- Auditory muscles
- Eustachian tube.

Auditory Ossicles

They are three minute bones:
1. Malleus
2. Incus
3. Stapes

Ossicles in the middle ear are attached to each other by ligaments. The handle of malleus is attached to tympanic membrane, and the foot plate of stapes lies in the oval window in the internal ear. When the sound waves strike the tympanic membrane these ossicles vibrate as a single unit.

Muscles

- Tensor tympani
- Stapedius.

Tensor Tympani

Function

Tensor tympani pulls and keeps the tympanic membrane tensed. Due to this vibrations on any portion of the tympanic membrane are transmitted to the malleus.

Stapedius

Function

Stapedius muscle prevents excess movements of the stapes.

Eustachian tube

Eustachian tube or the auditory tube extends from the middle ear to the nasopharynx.

It connects the middle ear to the posteriors part of the nose. It forms passage of air between the middle ear and atmosphere and equalizes pressure on both side of tympanic membrane.

Functions of Middle Ear

1. Transmission of sound from external ear through the ossicles to the middle ear.
2. Attenuation of sound by attenuation reflex.

Attenuation/tympanic reflex

It protects the tympanic membrane from being ruptured by loud sound and also protects the cochlea from damage by loud sound.

The reflex involves involuntary contraction of tensor tympani and stapedius muscles in response to a loud noise.

Internal Ear

The internal ear or labyrinth is a membranous structure enclosed by a bony labyrinth in petrous part of temporal bone.

It consists of:

- Cochlea—sense organ for hearing
- Vestibular apparatus—sense organ for equilibrium.

Cochlea

Cochlea is a coiled bony tube like snail's shell having two parts:

1. Central bony pillar called modiolus which has internal auditory canal with auditory nerve.
2. Bony canal which winds around the modiolus for two and a half times.

Compartments of Cochlea

Two membranes divide the spiral canal of cochlea into three compartments.

These membranes are:

- Basilar membrane
- Vestibular membrane

The components of cochlea are:

- Scala vestibuli.
- Scala tympani.
- Scala media.

All the three compartments are filled with fluid. Scala vestibuli and scala tympani contain perilymph, whereas the scala media contains endolymph.

Organ of Corti

Organ of Corti is the receptor organ for hearing. It rests upon the basilar membrane. The organ of Corti consists of supporting cells and receptors cells (inner and outer hair cells). These hair cells are supplied by network of cochlear nerve endings. They lead to spiral ganglion presents in modiolus.

Auditory pathway (Figs 10.6 and 10.7)

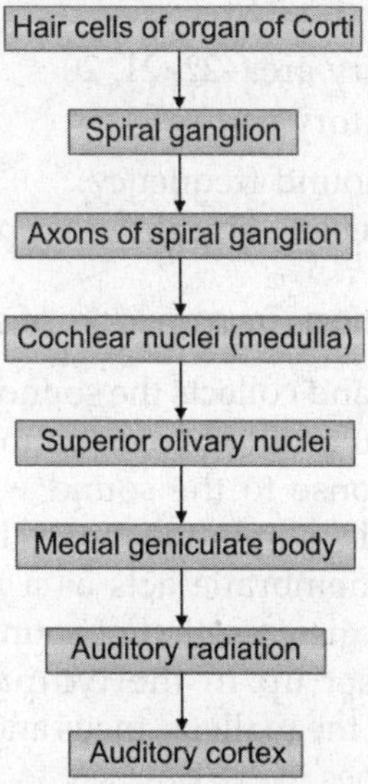

Fig. 10.6: Schematic flow diagram of auditory pathway

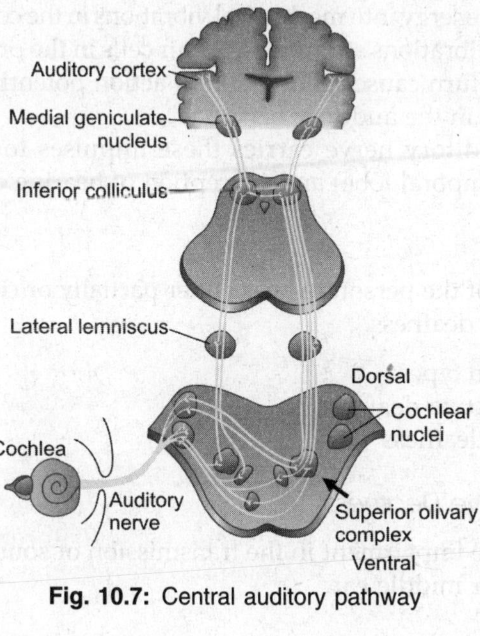

Fig. 10.7: Central auditory pathway

- Auditory cortex is present in the temporal lobe.
- Primary auditory area–41
- Secondary auditory area–22, 21, 20
- Functions of auditory cortex:
  - Perception of sound frequency.
  - Analysis of intensity and different properties of sound.

Mechanism of Hearing (Transmission of sound waves)

External ear detects and collects the sound waves, which travel through the external auditory meatus towards the tympanic membrane. In response to the sound waves on its external surface, the tympanic membrane moves in and out.

Thus tympanic membrane acts as a resonator and stops vibrating soon after the cessation of sound.

The vibrations set up in the tympanic membrane are transmitted through the malleus, incus and the stapes resulting in movement of stapes.

The movement of stapes produces vibrations in the fluids of cochlea. The tympanic membrane and auditory ossicles convert the sound energy into mechanical vibrations in the cochlear fluid.

These vibrations stimulate the hair cells in the organ of corti.

This is turn causes generation of action potential (auditory impulses) in the auditory nerve.

The auditory nerve carries these impulses to the central cortex (temporal lobe) and perception of hearing occurs.

Deafness

Inability of the person to hear either partially or completely is known as deafness.

It is of two types:
- Conductive deafness
- Nerve deafness

Conductive Deafness

It is due to impairment in the transmission of sound waves in external or middle ear.

Causes

- Foreign body or wax.
- Otitis media.
- Otosclerosis

Nerve Deafness

It is caused due to loss of function of organ of Corti or lesion in the auditory pathway.

Causes

- Toxic action of drugs like quinine, streptomycin.
- Trauma
- Tumor affecting VIII nerve.

Tests done for hearing

- Rinne's test
- Weber's test
- Audiometry

Review Questions

1. Write in brief about the mechanism of hearing
2. Describe in short the auditory pathway.
3. Define deafness. What are the different types of deafness? Mention the tests for deafness.
4. Write short notes on:
   - Functions of external ear
   - Functions of middle ear.
   - Attenuation reflex.

TASTE

The senses of taste and smell are closely interrelated and they are concerned mainly with nutrition.

Taste Buds

Tongue is concerned with taste sensation. Sense organs are the taste buds which contain hairs cells known as taste cells.

Taste buds are present on the tongue, palate, tonsillar pillars, and epiglottis and even on proximal oesophagus.

Structure of Taste Buds

- Taste buds consist of 7 to 10 taste cells and supporting cells.
- The taste cells have hair like projections called microvilli.
- The microvilli projects into an opening in the epithelium covering the tongue. This opening is called taste pore.

Pathway for Taste Sensations

Taste sensation is carried:

- From anterior two-thirds of tongue by facial nerve (VII)
- From the posterior one-third of tongue by glossopharyngeal (IX) nerve.

These nerve fibres carry the taste sensation to nucleus of tractus solitarius, from there to thalamus and finally relay in the parietal lobe of cerebral cortex.

Primary Taste Sensations (Fig. 10.8)

The primary fundamental taste sensations are sour, salty, sweet and bitter.

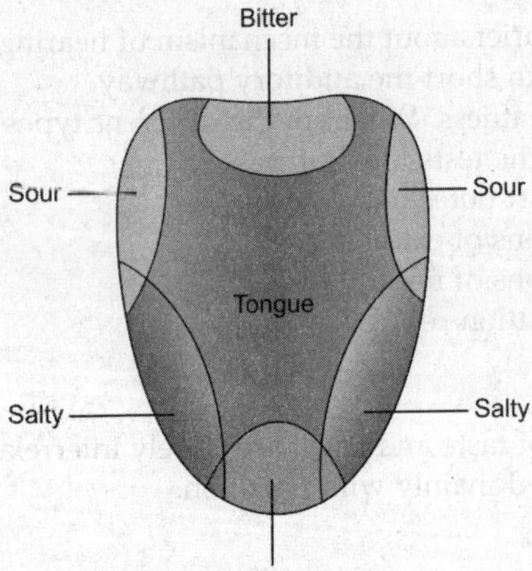

Fig. 10.8: Primary taste sensation

Recently umami is recognized as taste sensation. This taste sensation responds to glutamate as present in chinese food (Table 10.1).

Table 10.1: Taste sensation

Taste sensation	Chemical
Sweet	Monosaccharides, glycerol, alcohol, aldehydes, ketones.
Salt	Chlorides of sodium, potassium
Sour	Hydrogen ions in acids
Bitter	Quinine, strychnine, bile salts.

Mechanism of Taste Sensation

Taste is a chemical sense. Substance can be tasted only when it gets dissolved in saliva. The dissolved substance acts on the microvilli of taste receptor present in the taste pore which causes development of receptor potential. This is responsible for the generation of action potential in the sensory neurons.

Applied

Ageusia: Loss of taste sensation.
Hypogeusia: Decrease in the taste sensation.

Review Question

Write in brief about taste sensation.

SMELL

Olfactory Receptors

Receptors for smell sensation are olfactory cells. They lie in the olfactory epithelium present at the roof of the each nostril. The olfactory receptor cell is a bipolar neuron. The mucosal end of olfactory cell (dendrite) forms a knob called olfactory vesicle which contains tuft of cilia. The cilia project to the surface of olfactory epithelium.

Classification of Odor

Odor is classified into various types:
- Aromatic: Camphor, lavender
- Fragrant: Flowers, perfumes.
- Garlic: Garlic, onion
- Ethereal odor: Ether, fruits
- Burning: Tobacco.

Mechanism of Stimulation of Olfactory Cells

The odoriferous substance stimulates the olfactory receptors, after getting dissolved in mucus secreted by olfactory mucous membrane. Odorant materials bind to protein molecules present in the cilia causing opening of sodium channels and generating receptor potential. The action potential then travels in the axon of bipolar neuron.

Olfactory Pathway

Axons of bipolar cells form the olfactory nerves and pierce cribriform plate to reach olfactory bulb. From the olfactory bulb, olfactory tract runs backwards and ends in the olfactory cortex.

Applied

- **Anosmia**
  - Anosmia refers to total loss of sensation of smell
  - Like in common cold, nasal sinus.
- **Hyposmia:** Reduced ability to recognize odor.

Review Question

Write a note on sensation of smell.

11 Nervous System

ORGANIZATION OF NERVOUS SYSTEM

Nervous system controls all the activities of the body. The nervous system is divided into two main systems:

1. Central nervous system.
2. Peripheral nervous system.

Central Nervous System

Central nervous system includes brain and spinal cord. It is formed by neurons and supporting cells called neuroglia. Nervous system is comprised white and gray matter (Fig. 11.1).

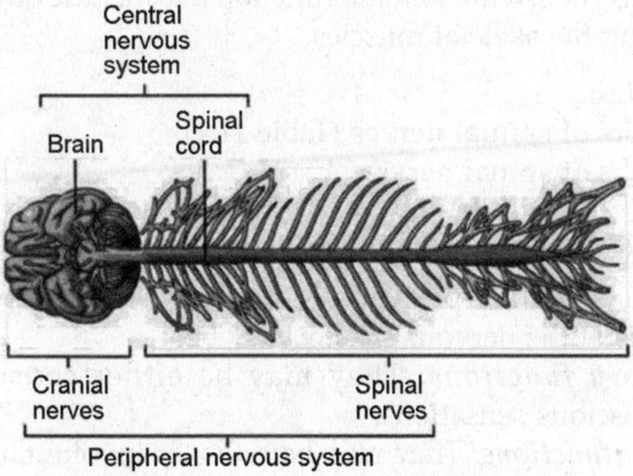

Fig. 11.1: Central nervous system

The gray matter is formed by nerve cell bodies and proximal part of the nerve fibres arising from the nerve cell body whereas white matter is formed by nerve fibres.

In brain the white matter is present centrally and gray matter outside. In spinal cord white matter is the outer part and gray matter in the inner part.

The brain and spinal cord are surrounded by three layers of meninges, the outer dura mater, middle arachnoid and inner pia mater

The brain and spinal cord are suspended in the cerebrospinal fluid.

Peripheral Nervous System

It is divided into two subdivision:

1. Somatic nervous system.
2. Autonomic nervous system.

Autonomic Nervous System

It is concerned with regulation of visceral or vegetative functions. It is divided into two subdivision sympathetic division and parasympathetic division.

Somatic Nervous System

It is concerned with somatic functions. It includes the nerves supplying the skeletal muscles.

It includes:

- 12 pairs of **cranial nerves** (Table 11.1)
- 31 pairs of **spinal nerves**.

General Functions of Nervous System

Depending on the type of nerve impulse and its interpretation, functions of the nervous system may be:

1. ***Sensory functions:*** They may be either conscious or unconscious sensations.
2. ***Motor functions:*** They may be reflex or involuntary.
3. ***Associative functions:*** For instance, memory, intelligence, idea, etc.

Review Questions

1. How is nervous system classified?
2. Enumerates the cranial nerves.

Nerves	Type	Function
1. Olfactory	sensory	olfaction (smell)
2. Optic	sensory	vision
3. Oculomotor	motor	eyelid and eyeball muscles
4. Trochlear	motor	eyeball muscles
5. Trigeminal	mixed	Sensory: Facial and mouth sensation Motor: Chewing
6. Abducens	motor	eyeball movement
7. Facial	mixed	Sensory: Taste Motor: Facial muscles and salivary glands
8. Auditory	sensory	hearing and balance
9. Glossopharyngeal	mixed	Sensory: Taste Motor: Swallowing
10. Vagus	mixed	main nerve of the parasympathetic nervous system (PNS)
11. Accessory	motor	swallowing; moving head and shoulder
12. Hypoglossal	motor	tongue muscles

Table 11.1: The cranial nerves

BRAIN (Figs 11.2 and 11.3)

Brain consists of three major divisions:

- Prosencephalon (forebrain).
- Mesencephalon (midbrain).
- Rhombencephalon (hindbrain).

Cerebral Cortex

Cerebrum consists of two symmetrical hemispheres connected by corpus callosum. The total surface area of adult cortex is about 2200 sq.cm. Each hemisphere has four main lobes (Fig. 11.3).

1. Frontal lobe.
2. Parietal lobe.
3. Temporal lobe.
4. Occipital lobe.

Frontal Lobe

It is present in front of the precentral gyrus. It includes the precentral cortex (pre motor area, areas 4, 6, 8, 44) and prefrontal

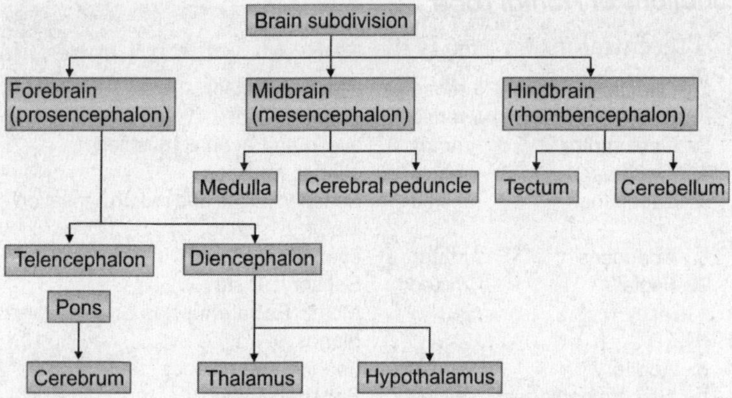

Fig. 11.2: Brain subdivision

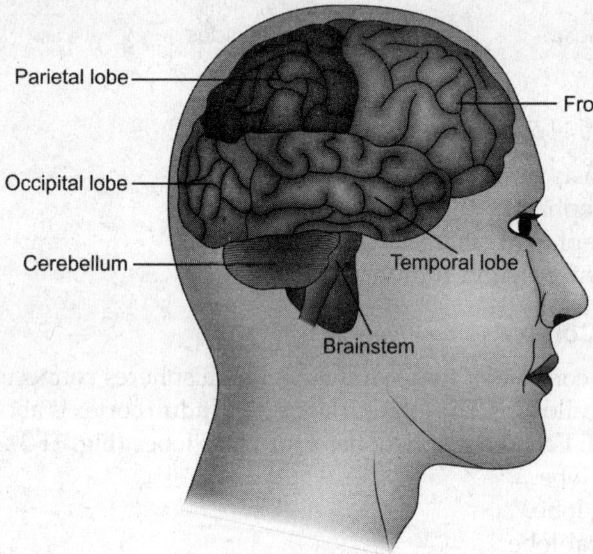

Fig. 11.3: Lobes of brain

cortex (areas 9, 10, 11, 12, 32). The pre frontal lobe is the anterior part of the cerebrum.

Functions of Frontal Lobe

- Precentral motor area is the centre for volition. Centres for the various parts of the body are arranged upside down.
- It helps in controlling complex movements of jaws, tongue, pharynx, larynx, swallowing and also the activity of respiratory muscles.
- It contains Broca's area (area 44) which is the centre for speech.
- It contains area 8 (frontal eye field), which controls the conjugate movements of eyeball to the opposite side.
- The prefrontal lobe is the seat of intelligence.
- Prefrontal lobe helps in complex intellectual activities like, giving judgment, solving mathematical problems, etc.
- Prefrontal lobe through their connections with hypothalamus exerts their influence on autonomic nervous system.
- It is also concerned with memory, emotions social and moral behavior.

Due to its functions prefrontal lobe is also known as ***Organ of mind.***

Frontal Lobe Syndrome

Lesions in the prefrontal lobe is called frontal lobe syndrome.

The symptoms are:
- Lack of initiative.
- Lack of self-control.
- Difficulty of attention.
- Impairment of moral and social sense.
- Euphoria.
- Loss of memory.

Parietal Lobe

It is present behind the postcentral gyrus and includes sensory area (somaesthetic area or primary sensory area, areas 3, 1, 2) and sensory association area (areas 5, 7).

Functions of Parietal Lobe

- Appreciation of general senses, such as heat, cold, pain and kinaesthetic from the opposite side of the body.
- Appreciation of size, shape, texture of the objects—stereognosis.

- Tactile localization, tactile discrimination.
- The association areas help to understand and interpret the sensory stimuli.

Damage of the parietal lobe leads to

1. *Agnosia:* Failure to recognize own body part.
2. *Aphasia:* Speech disturbance.
3. Astereognosis.

Temporal Lobe

It includes sensory (auditosensory area, area 41) and association area (auditopsychic area, areas 22, 21, 20).

Functions of Temporal Lobe

- Auditosensory area is the centre for hearing. Here the pitch, loudness, quality of the sounds is perceived.
- Association areas analyze, interpret and integrate the auditory impulses. It is thus related to speech and language functions.
- It is also involved in olfaction.

Lesions of the temporal lobe leads to abnormalities like:

- Poor memory.
- Speech disorder.
- Auditory disturbances.
- Psychomotor epilepsy.

Occipital Lobe

This part of the brain is involved in vision. It includes the sensory (visuosensory area, area 17) and association area (visuopsychic area, areas 18, 19).

Functions of Occipital Lobe

- Visuosensory area is the visual centre.
- It receives and recognizes visual information including colors, feature, and movement.
- Association area helps in understanding the exact meaning of visual image.

- Lesions of the occipital cortex lead to various types of visual abnormalities. Person with lesion in this area will fail to understand the meaning of written language.

Summarization of important areas of cerebral cortex (Brodmann's areas)

1. *Primary motor area (area 4):* It is in the precentral gyrus and is responsible for execution of movements.
2. *Premotor area (areas 6 and 8):* It contributes motor fibres to both pyramidal and extrapyramidal pathways. It is involved in coordination and programming of movements (Figs 11.4a and b).

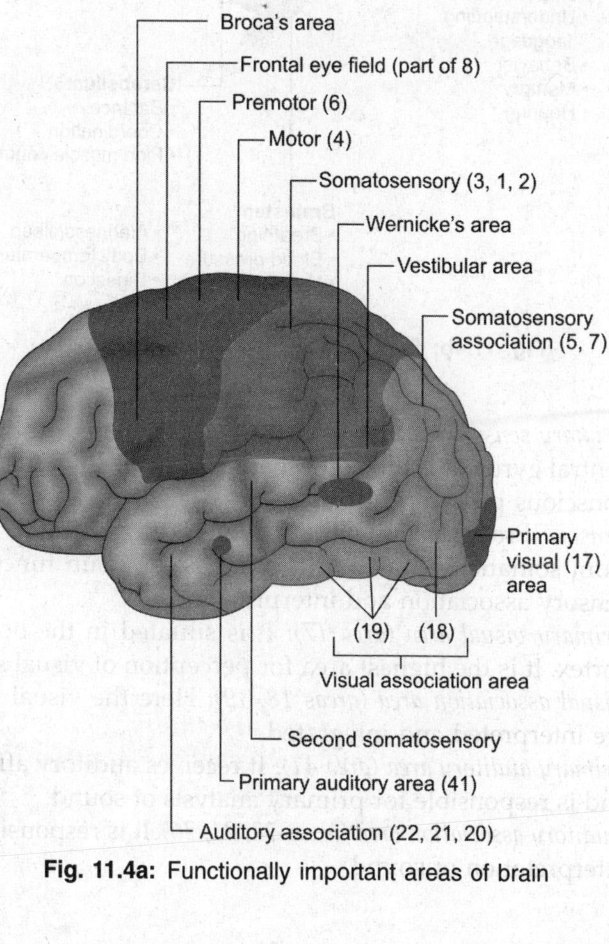

Fig. 11.4a: Functionally important areas of brain

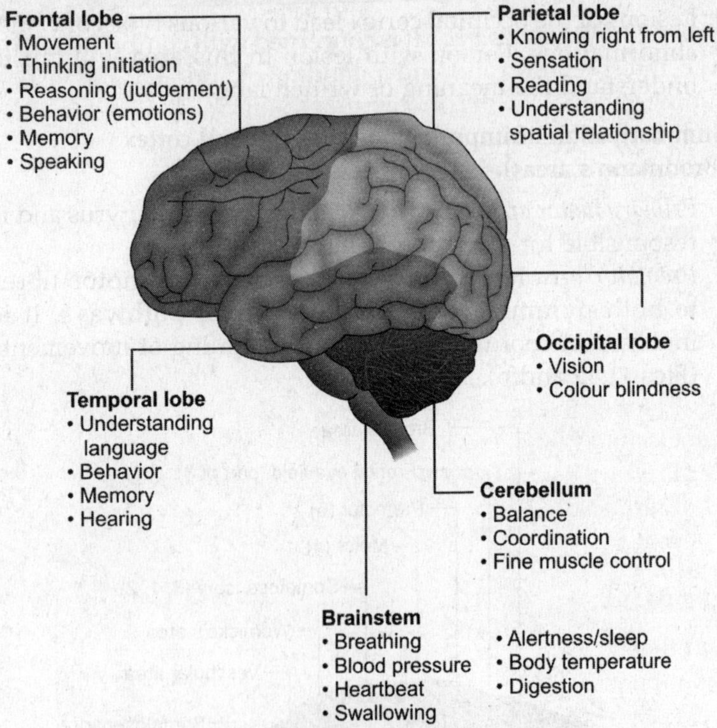

Fig. 11.4b: Functionally important areas of brain

3. *Primary sensory area (areas 3, 1, 2):* It is situated in the post central gyrus. It is the highest area for the somaesthetic and conscious proprioceptive senses.
4. *Sensory association area (areas 5, 7):* It receives sensory inputs from somatic, visual, auditory areas. Its main function is sensory association and interpretation.
5. *Primary visual area (area 17):* It is situated in the occipital cortex. It is the highest area for perception of visual sense.
6. *Visual association area (areas 18, 19):* Here the visual senses are interpreted and integrated.
7. *Primary auditory area (area 41):* It receives auditory afferents and is responsible for primary analysis of sound.
8. *Auditory association area (areas 22, 21, 20):* It is responsible for interpretation of sound.

9. *Area 22 (Wernicke's area):* It is concerned with comprehension, i.e. interpretation and understanding of auditory and visual information. Damage to this area results in sensory aphasia, i.e. the patient cannot understand the meaning of heard as well as written words.

Review Questions

1. Give the divisions of brain.
2. Write short notes on:
   a. Parietal lobe.
   b. Frontal lobe.
   c. Temporal lobe.
   d. Occipital lobe.
   e. Prefrontal syndrome.
   f. Enumerate the functionally important areas of cerebral cortex.

HYPOTHALAMUS

Hypothalamus is a diencephalic structure situated below the thalamus.

Functions

Though hypothalamus constitutes only 1% of the brain mass, it deals with many important functions:

1. Secretion of posterior pituitary hormones like, antidiuretic (ADH) and oxytocin.
2. Anterior pituitary functions:
   a. By secreting various releasing hormones, hypothalamus controls the secretion of anterior pituitary.
   b. Growth hormone releasing hormone (GHRH).
   c. Thyrotropin releasing hormone (TRH).
   d. Corticotropin releasing hormone (CRH).
   e. Gonadotropin releasing hormone (GnRH).
3. It helps in the regulation of body temperature.
4. It helps in regulation of water balance.
5. It helps in regulation of hunger and food intake.
6. It helps in cardiovascular regulation by regulating heart rate and blood pressure.

7. It has role in behavioral and emotional functions.
8. It maintains the circadian rhythm.

BASAL GANGLIA

Basal ganglia are the group of nuclei present at the base of cerebral cortex.

The basal ganglia includes:
1. Corpus striatum which includes caudate nucleus and lenticular nucleus.
2. Subthalamic nucleus.
3. Substantia nigra.

Functions

1. Voluntary motor activity
   - The movements during voluntary motor activity are initiated by the cerebral cortex but are controlled by basal ganglia.
   - It regulates semiautomatic movements like swinging of arms during walking, movements of limbs during swimming.
2. *Control of reflex muscular activity:* Basal ganglia exert inhibitory effect on spinal reflexes and regulate activity of muscles which maintains posture.
3. It also controls muscle tone.

Applied

Parkinson's disease

The Parkinson's disease is a slowly progressive degenerative disease associated with damage of dopamine producing cells of basal ganglia. It is mostly due to destruction of substantia nigra.

Signs and Symptoms

1. Tremor.
2. Slowness of movements.
3. Poverty of movements.
4. Rigidity.
5. Speech problems.

6. Festinant gate.
7. Emotional changes.
8. Dementia.

THALAMUS

Thalamus is an egg shaped mass of grey matter situated bilaterally in diencephalon.

Functions

Functionally, thalamus represents the coordinate centre where sensory, motor and autonomic information can be brought together to produce harmonious activity.

The various functions of thalamus are:

1. ***Relay station:*** Thalamus forms the relay centre for pathways coming from cerebellum, cerebral cortex, and peripheral nervous system.
2. It is a major centre for processing the sensory information as well as determining the quality of sensations.
3. Because of intimate connections between thalamus, frontal cortex and hypothalamus, it is involved in subjective feeling of emotions.
4. Thalamus has a role in arousal and alerting reactions.
5. Thalamus also serves as a centre for integration of motor functions.

THALAMIC SYNDROME

It is a condition produced due to damage and resultant defective functions of thalamus. Following features are seen in thalamic syndrome:

- Sensations from the opposite side of the body are diminished.
- Sensory ataxia.
- Thalamic phantom limb.
- Motor disturbances like abnormal movements, and tremor.

THE CEREBELLUM

Cerebellum is the largest part of the hindbrain and lies in the posterior (occipital) fossa.

It is made up of two cerebellar hemispheres joined by vermis.

Functionally it has following subdivisions:
- Vestibulocerebellum.
- Spinocerebellum.
- Neocerebellum.

Functions of Cerebellum

- Vestibulocerebellum helps in the regulation of posture and equilibrium.
- Spinocerebellum helps in regulation of muscle tone.
- Neocerebellum is concerned with integration and regulation of coordinated muscular activities, so that the movements may be accurate in time, force, direction and extent.
- Cerebellum does not initiate any motor activity but assists the action initiated by the cortex.
- Cerebellum helps in the control of ballistic movements. Ballistic movements are rapid alternate movements which takes place in different parts of the body while doing skilled work like typing, dancing.

Cerebellar Lesions

Common causes of cerebellar damage are:
- Tumor.
- Injury.
- Thrombosis of the artery supplying cerebellum.

Sign and Symptoms

- Hypotonia.
- Ataxia.
- Asthenia.
- Past pointing.
- Intention tremor.
- Scanning speech.
- Adiadochokinesis.
- Dysmetria.

Review Questions

1. Write down the functions of thalamus.
2. Mention in brief the role of hypothalamus in body.
3. Give the functions of basal ganglia.

4. Write in brief the function of cerebellum. Add a note on cerebellar lesions.
5. Write short notes on:
   a. Thalamic syndrome.
   b. Parkinson's disease.

SENSORY SYSTEM

Sensations

Definition: Sensations are feelings aroused by change of environment.

Classification of Sensations

Sensations are classified as:
- General.
- Special senses–vision hearing, smell and taste.

General Senses

General sensations are divided further into:
Superficial deep and visceral.
1. *Superficial*: They arise from skin. They are of two types: epicretic and protopathic sensations.
   a. *Epicretic:* The mild or light sensations are epicretic sensations, e.g. fine touch, tactile localization, and tactile discrimination.
   b. *Protopathic:* The crude part of the various cutaneous sensations is protopathic sensations, e.g. pressure, temperature, pain.
2. *Deep sensations:* They arise from deep structures, e.g. deep pain, vibration sense, kinaesthetic sense (ability to recognize degree of movement and position of muscles and limb).
3. *Visceral sensations:* They arise from the viscera, e.g. distension of stomach, bladder, visceral pain.

Components of Sensory System

The sensory system comprises the following:
- Receptor.
- Neural pathway (tracts).
- Somatosensory cortex.

Receptors

Definition: Receptor is a modified sensory nerve ending which undergoes depolarization in response to a specific stimulus and sends information to the central nervous system. It is also called as biological transducer that converts various forms of energy into electrical energy (action potential) (Fig. 11.5).

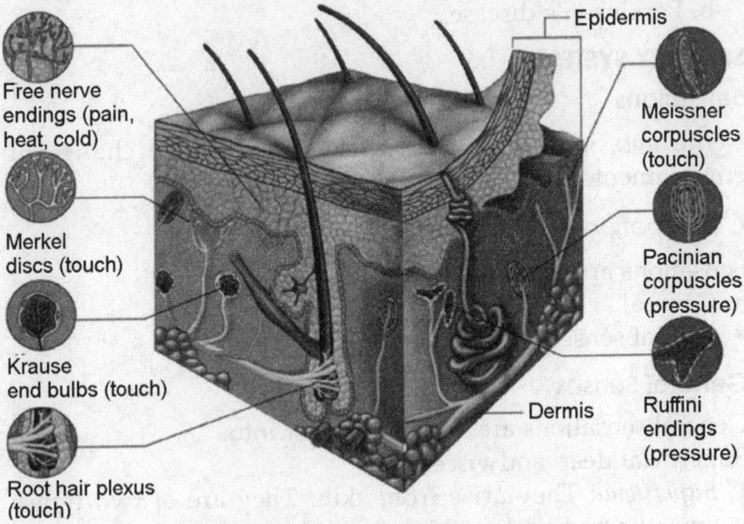

Fig. 11.5: Sensory receptors in skin

Classification of Receptors

- *Mechanoreceptors:* Touch, pressure.
- *Chemoreceptors:* Taste, smell.
- *Thermal receptors:* Warmth, cold.
- *Electromagnetic receptors:* Rods and cones.
- *Nociceptors:* Pain nerve endings.

General Senses

A. **Cutaneous endings for superficial sensation.**
- *For touch:* Meissner's corpuscles, Merkel's disc.
- *For deep pressure:* Pacinian corpuscles.
- For heat-end organs of Golgi and Ruffini.
- For pain-free nerve endings.

B. **Deep endings for kinaesthetic/proprioceptive sensations.** Proprioceptors of muscles, tendons and joints-muscle spindle, Golgi tendon organ.

NEURAL PATHWAY

These are the ascending tract (sensory tracts) in the spinal cord (Table 11.2)

Table 11.2: Sensory tracts and functions

Tracts	*Functions*
Tract of Goll (fasiculus gracilis)	Fine touch, tactile localization. Discrimination, kinaesthetic sensation,Vibration sensation from the lower half of the body.
Tract of Burdach (fasciculus cuneatus)	Carries same sensations from the upper half of the body.
Lateral spinothalamic tract	Pain and temperature
Ventral spinothalamic tract	Touch and tactile localization
Spinocerebellar tract	Unconscious kinaesthetic sensation

Somatosensory Cortex

It lies in the parietal lobe. It includes primary sensory area (areas 3, 1, 2) and association area (areas 5, 7) (Fig. 11.6).

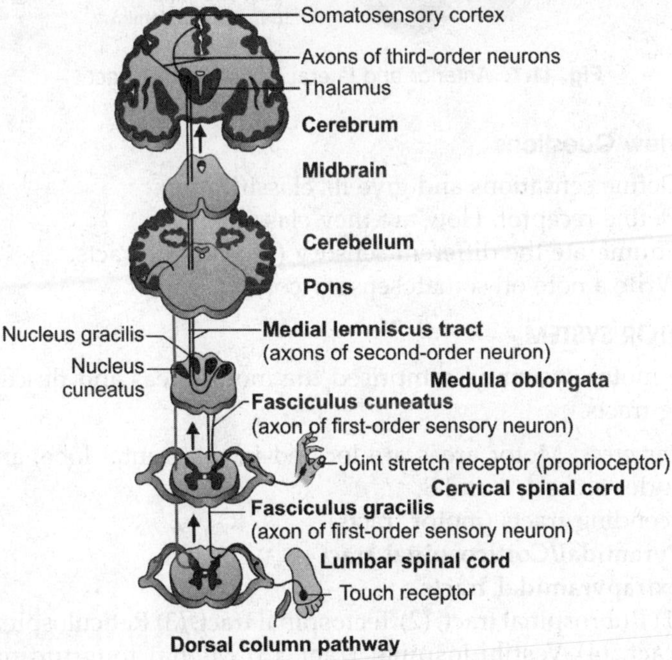

Fig. 11.6: Tractus gracilis and cuneatus

Spinothalamic Tract (Fig. 11.7)

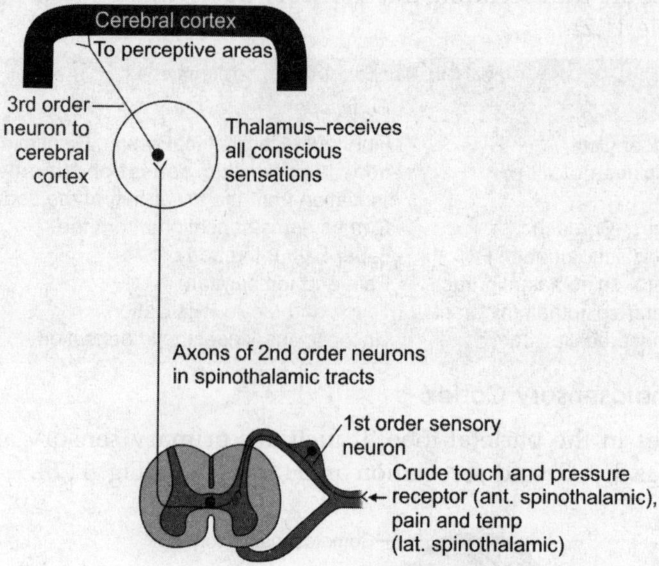

Fig. 11.7: Anterior and lateral spinothalamic tract

Review Questions

1. Define sensations and give its classification.
2. Define receptor. How are they classified?
3. Enumerate the different sensory (ascending) tracts.
4. Write a note on somatosensory cortex.

MOTOR SYSTEM

The motor system is comprised the motor areas and descending tracts.

Motor areas: Motor areas are located in the frontal lobe, and includes areas 4, 6 and 8.

Descending tracts (motor tracts).

A. **Pyramidal/Corticospinal tract**

B. **Extrapyramidal tracts**

(1) Rubrospinal tract, (2) Tectospinal tract, (3) Reticulospinal tract, (4) Vestibulospinal tract, (5) Medial longitudinal fasciculus.

Pyramidal Tract

The fibres of the pyramidal tract arise from the motor and somatosensory areas of cerebral cortex.

The fibres after originating pass through the internal capsule, midbrain, pons, medulla and finally end in the motor neurons of anterior gray horn of spinal cord. The axons of the motor neurons leave spinal cord as spinal nerves and supply the skeletal muscles.

Functions of Pyramidal Tract

The pyramidal tract plays a role in controlling the voluntary movements, especially of fingers and hands in performance of skilled work (Fig. 11.8).

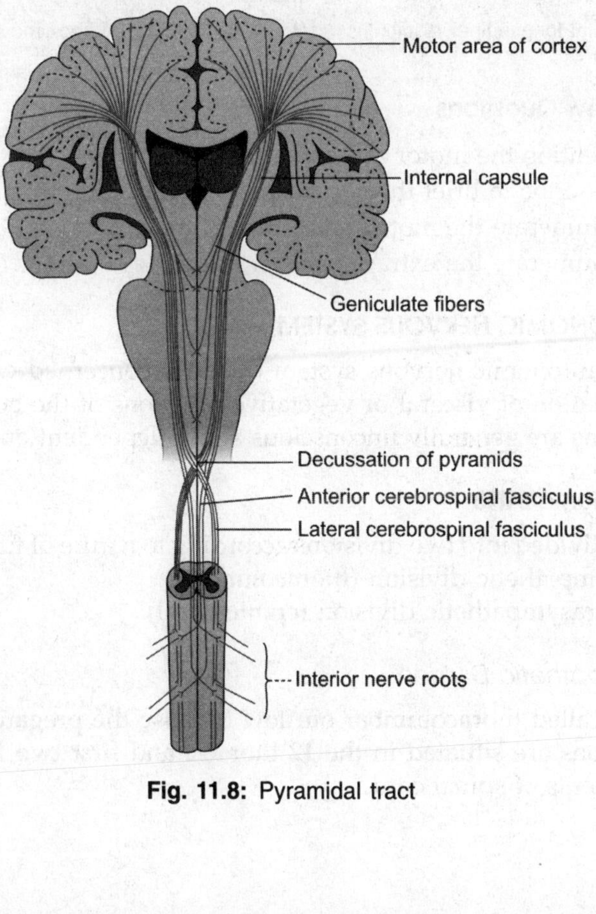

Fig. 11.8: Pyramidal tract

Extrapyramidal Tracts

The descending tracts other than pyramidal tract which are also involved in muscle movement and posture are called extrapyramidal tracts (Table 11.3).

Table 11.3: Extrapyramidal tract and its functions

Tract	*Function*
Rubrospinal tract	It has a facilitatory influence over flexor muscle tone
Tectospinal tract	Help in postural movements in response to visual and auditory stimuli
Reticulospinal tract	Control of muscle tone, control of blood pressure and respiration
Vestibulospinal tract	Facilitatory influence over antigravity muscles.
Medial longitudinal fasciculus	Integration of eye and neck movements

Review Questions

1. Mention the motor areas and their functions.
2. Describe in brief the corticospinal (pyramidal) tract.
3. Enumerate the motor (descending) tracts.
4. Enumerate the extrapyramidal tracts.

AUTONOMIC NERVOUS SYSTEM (ANS)

The autonomic nervous system (ANS) is concerned with the regulation of visceral or vegetative functions of the body. Its actions are generally unconscious and independent on *will*.

Division of ANS

It is divided into two divisions according to nature of function:
- Sympathetic division (thoracolumbar).
- Parasympathetic division (craniosacral).

Sympathetic Division

It is called thoracolumbar outflow because the preganglionic neurons are situated in the 12 thoracic and first two lumbar segments of spinal cord.

Sympathetic division supplies smooth muscle fibres of all the visceral organs such as blood vessels, heart, lungs, gastro-intestinal organs, glands, etc.

Parasympathetic Division

The parasympathetic division of ANS is called craniosacral outflow since the fibres of this division arise from brain and sacral segments of spinal cord. The cranial portion of parasympathetic division innervates blood vessels of head, neck and many thoracoabdominal visceral organs.

The sacral portion in sacral segments innervates the smooth muscles of viscera such as large intestine, liver, spleen, kidneys, bladder, etc. (Fig. 11.9).

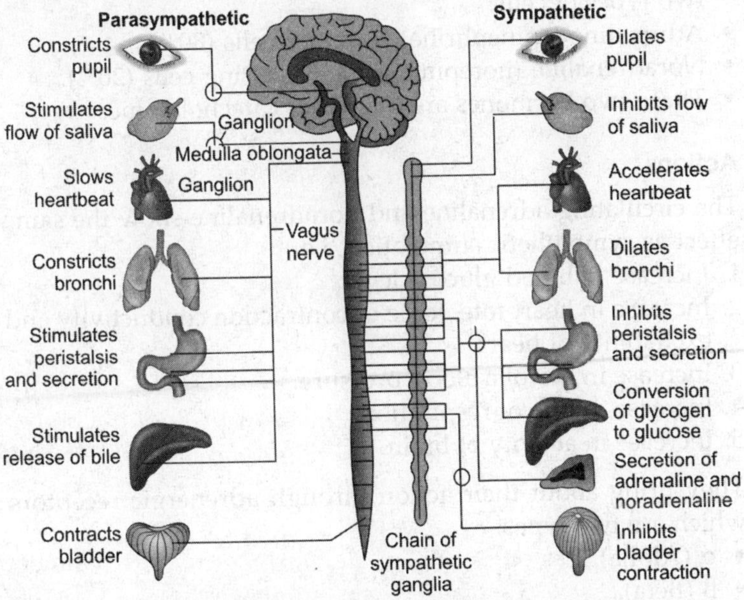

Fig. 11.9: Functions of sympathetic and parasympathetic nervous system

Function of ANS

It regulates the activity of smooth muscles, heart, glands of GIT, sweat glands, adrenal glands and endocrine glands automatically.

It is known as involuntary or vegetative nervous system (vegetative because concerned with growth and day-to-day living).

In summary, the sympathetic and parasympathetic system, by acting oppositely helps in maintaining optimal internal environment of the body.

The nerve fibres of ANS execute the function by releasing some neurotransmitter substances.

Sympathetic fibres secrete—noradrenaline
Parasympathetic fibres secrete–acetylcholine

Adrenal Medulla

- Medulla is the inner part of the adrenal gland. It consists of two types of cells:
- Adrenaline (epinephrine) secreting cells (80%).
- Noradrenaline (norepinephrine) secreting cells (20%).
- These two hormones are known as catecholamines.

Actions

The circulating adrenaline and noradrenaline show the same effect as sympathetic stimulation, i.e.

1. Increase in blood glucose level.
2. Increase in heart rate, force of contraction conductivity and excitability of heart.
3. Increase in systolic blood pressure.
4. Increase in rate of respiration.
5. Increase in activity of brain.

They bring about their action through adrenergic receptors which are two types:

- α (Alpha).
- β (Beta).

Review Questions

1. Write in brief on autonomic nervous system.
2. Enumerate the functions of autonomic nervous system.

Index